FREE YOUR SPIRIT WITH MOVEMENT

In the workplace and at home, we relentlessly drive ourselves to "produce," every day of every month, year after year. Now, many women are beginning to ask, "For what?" As we grow older and the external world becomes ever more stressful, our bodies sometimes seem to turn on us—just when we most need balance and stability.

If you're like many women, you've somehow lost the connection between your spirit, intellect, and body. As you have moved into middle age, you may have begun searching for a way to heal the imbalance you feel in your life. But you don't know what that process involves—or even how to get started.

Come Home to Your Body is a workbook that will guide you through the process of raising your body awareness and reconnecting with your spirit—through movement.

Perform simple, yet profound, exercises that will help you feel the vibrant dance of energy running through you at every moment. You'll learn to stay centered in inner peace and power, even during stressful, hectic times. To release blocks to your energy flow and prevent chronic pain by being aware of your body's changing comfort levels. To move freely and painlessly your entire life, whatever your age. Finally, you'll regain your birthright: an organic connection with your spirit and inner wisdom.

Many of us are discovering we have lost a crucial connection with our bodies. The process of "coming home to your body" is to understand that you are your body, with a wisdom far deeper than that of your intellect. Stop ignoring that wisdom. Come home to your body and find the peace of mind, physical comfort, and connection with your spirit you've been yearning for ... they await you within.

LLEWELLYN'S WHOLE LIFE SERIES

COME HOME

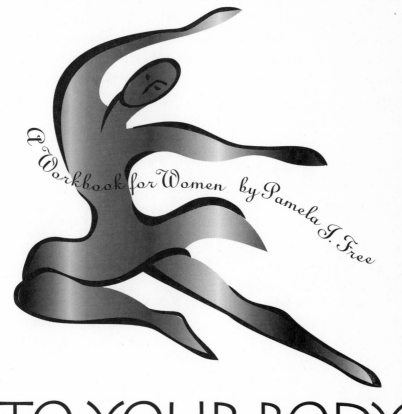

A Workbook for Women by Pamela J. Free

TO YOUR BODY

1997
LLEWELLYN PUBLICATIONS
ST. PAUL, MINNESOTA, 55164-0383, U.S.A.

FIRST EDITION
First Printing, 1996

Cover art and design: Anne Marie Garrison
Book editing, design, and layout: Deb Gruebele
Project coordination: Connie Hill
Interior art, pp. 34–35: Pamela J. Free

Library of Congress Cataloging-in-Publication Data

Free, Pamela J., 1944–
    Come Home to your body : a workbook for women / Pamela J. Free. —
1st ed.
        p.   cm. — (Llewellyn's whole life series)
    ISBN 1-56718-290-9
    1. Feldenkrais method.   2. Women—Mental health.   3. Women—Health
and hygiene.   I. Title.   II. Series.
RC489.F44F74   1997   96-33511
613' .04244—dc20   CIP

Printed in the United States of America.

Llewellyn Publications
A Division of Llewellyn Worldwide, Ltd.
St. Paul, Minnesota, 55164-0383, U.S.A.

ABOUT LLEWELLYN'S WHOLE LIFE SERIES

Each of us is born into a body, but an amazing number of us lack anything beyond the most utilitarian connection with our physical beings. Yet, being "in touch" with the body—being aware of the senses' connection to our thoughts, emotions, dreams, and spirits—is integral to holistic living.

What does the physical have to do with the emotional or the spiritual? Everything. We are as much beings of the Earth as we are beings of the stars … our senses and connection to our bodies are just as integral to our physical, emotional, and spiritual well-being as is our connection to our higher selves.

The old doctrines, which regard the physical as inferior to the spiritual, may have made sense for the medieval ascetic—but, much like the medieval belief that the Sun orbited the Earth, those beliefs have been supplanted by more enlightened ones. Fortunately. Because it is impossible to truly feel that we belong in the universe, just as much as the ground we walk on and the air we breathe, until we entirely accept our own natures as physical and spiritual creatures. This book will help you heal the split between will and understanding, and further your journey to wholeness, the place where body, mind, and spirit are integrated and healed. Access your internal source of wisdom, love, and healing through the techniques presented here for heightened mind and body awareness … and become so much more than the sum of your parts.

COMING HOME TO MY BODY

As a child, I tumbled and twirled,
danced, walked on my hands,
swung upside down from iron railings,
did headstands, handstands, cartwheels.
Dreamed of joining the circus, flying on a trapeze.
"Don't pay her any mind," said my sister, Diana,
"she can't help it, she's double-jointed."

Then came puberty, red blood flowing, strange and unexpected.
Keep my knees together, keep my feet on the floor,
grow up, act my age, behave myself,
walk like a lady, sit up straight,
everyone is looking at me, I'm not doing it right.
Shame, shame, shame.
I'll just leave my body.

I missed so many years of the rhythms of my body.
The ebbing and the flowing, the stretching and the growing,
all my systems circulating in their own mysterious patterns.
Muscles, glands, organs, blood and breath
all pulsing and oozing, squeezing and leaping.
Magical transitions from desire into impulse into movement.
One thought creating a trillion interactions in the patterns of my cells
leading to my arms going up or my feet going down.
Each time my hand reaches out for another
there occurs a miracle of so many dimensions,
energy and aura, muscle and bone, longing and yearning
all translating into simple action.
How could I have been absent for so long
from my own true self?

No time now for regret.
Only time to pay attention
to bring my awareness to the pleasure
of being the Prodigal Daughter
returned to my own loving arms.
The exquisite sensations of skin,
the languorous joy of muscles stretching,
the intensity of energy dancing.
Time to roll on the floor,
make circular movements,
explore, rejoice, experience, feel.
Come home to my body.

Pamela J. Free

To Caroline Conger,
who first inspired me with the deep and mysterious
power of the feminine.

TABLE OF CONTENTS

ACKNOWLEDGMENTS

My first thanks go to my mother, who has always been sure I can do anything, and to Yvette and Tim, who are my first line of loving support and who gave me the computer that made this book possible.

Then I thank all the women who have taught me, helped me, loved me, laughed with me over the years, rubbing gently away at all my sharp edges, my hasty judgments, and my impatience.

Next Judith, who said that I had to write a workbook; Shannon, Flavienne, Hari-nam, Petra, Connie, Lilli, Val, Katherine, Patty, Sharon, Peg, and all the members of my spiritual group; all my very special clients, many of whom became friends; all of the diverse and inspiring members of my Feldenkrais training group who rolled on the floor and learned and grew in strange and wonderful ways for four years. Much appreciation to Mara Gourley, who created the illustrations of women breathing. It was a collaboration that has led to loving sisterhood.

Lastly, my deep gratitude to all my various teachers along life's winding path. I have been truly blessed.

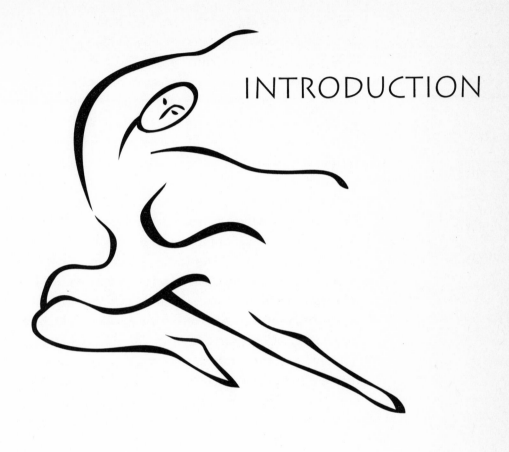

INTRODUCTION

This book grew out of my intensive work with women over the last fifteen years. I have watched a huge shift in consciousness over those years, in myself and in my clients, as both the world of women and the external world have changed so rapidly. I have heard the voices of women from all walks of life calling out for a way to correct the imbalance in their lives. Women are ready to recognize and acknowledge their yearning to regain contact with their bodies from the inside, to live from within their body wisdom, and by so doing, to wake up to their spirit. Body, mind, and spirit all must be connected and acknowledged in our daily lives for us to feel joy and inner peace, health and vitality. The current dominance of the mind over the body, and the ignoring of our spirituality, has created much disease and disharmony within us.

Many of us who were born, or grew up, in the fifties, joyfully embraced the revolutionary changes feminism brought to our lives. We sallied forth to find ourselves in the world of work, pursuing interesting and worthwhile careers. We were going to make our mark on the world. It was as if we had finally been invited to the prince's ball instead of staying home like Cinderella.

Now as we move into our forties, fifties, and sixties, it is beginning to dawn on us how much we lost in this transformation. It is obvious to most of us by now that we gave up essential parts of ourselves to fit into the male-dominated workplace. In our struggle to be accepted into that world, we have learned to think like men, putting aside our natural, intuitional, right-brained way of perceiving life. Mind became paramount, the only part of us with true, marketable value.

Meanwhile, back at the home front, it is well documented that our partners did not as eagerly embrace the dual roles of bread-winner and home-maker. What women actually did was exchange one primary role for two. As the word primary suggests, one role inevitably demanded more energy than the other, creating conflict that is not present in the lives of most men. Some of us decided that our career was primary and so our personal relationships suffered. Some of us put our work in the background and settled for boring, routine tasks. Some of us juggled back and forth, keeping all our balls in the air by moving faster and faster. What most of us gave up somewhere along the way was deep contact with our own bodies and with the spirit that animates the body.

I recently read, in a popular women's magazine, a list of directives for the New American Woman:

Be loved.
Think positive.
Eat right.
Stay fit.

Enrich your mind.

Save the World.

Doesn't it make you tired? Women in the '90s are already overloaded. This is a list of goals that comes directly from the left brain. It ignores the wonderful complexity of our lives and implies that if we work hard enough on all these fronts at once, we may eventually achieve success. We still have the pivotal role in the family as nurturer and care-giver, and too often as a single parent. Some of us are struggling with combining children from different marriages, yet most of us now need to earn at least part of the family income also.

We haven't *changed* our roles, we have *added* whole new lists of tasks to our job descriptions. Our internal taskmasters are taking responsibility for more and more. Our mothers and grandmothers didn't feel the need to make themselves responsible for the entire planet. Where does this list speak of our yearning for inner wholeness, for comfort in our body/mind, for connection to spirit, both our own and the larger Spirit of humankind?

For many of us now, our children are finally grown up and leaving home, many of them leaving later than any previous generation. Some of us have accumulated a significant amount of possessions from all these years of work, while others are still struggling financially. We all have our individual life dramas and special circumstances laying claim to our attention, but wherever women are gathered together, speaking from their hearts, I have heard a new willingness to stop and take stock of their lives in a meaningful way. We yearn for some sign of movement forward into the earned space of "Wise Woman," and dread instead the downward spiral into the dishonored role of "Old Woman." We look at our health and our sense of well-being and we often find it lacking.

Over the years of coping with too much work and too little time, the one part of our lives that could most easily be shoved aside was self-care, self-nurturing. We put everyone and everything ahead of our connection with ourselves. Most of us can

... wherever women are gathered together, speaking from their hearts, I have heard a new willingness to stop and take stock of their lives in a meaningful way.

look back over our years of raising a family or having a career or both, and see clearly how much of ourselves we have given up in order to be present for others.

When I ask my clients—"What do *you* want? What do *you* feel? What brings *you* pleasure?"—they struggle to find the answers. Giving themselves up has become a habit. They no longer notice that they do it. A client was planning to attend one of my workshops on coming home to your body, and she didn't show up. She explained later that her teenage son had needed a ride to a football game at the last minute. It didn't occur to her that her plans had any justifiable priority.

It is the premise of this book that it is only by taking care of *ourselves*, getting back in touch with our bodies and all the feelings that they store, and making time to integrate body, mind, and spirit, that we can ever hope to have the balance and resources to take care of others or to heal the world.

I would love to see a huge shift in women's consciousness in the next few years so that we can enter the new century with a more realistic and healthy regard for the importance of a woman's special place in this society. Society as a whole desperately needs more of the skills that come with the feminine side of our natures. We have sacrificed the expression of our feelings, and our needs for bonding and for community, and we have received less in return than can support us.

Now our work in the marketplace has become expected of us, and those women who choose to stay home and raise children find themselves apologizing for their lack of productivity or ambition. We have become commodities in a system that does not value our special skills and talents.

Our health has suffered as we have increasingly lost touch with our bodies. The wisdom of the body is seen as an intriguing new idea. The ebbs and flows of life that live in the body— day and night, spring and fall, hormonal cycles, birthing, maturing, and growing older—all have been forgotten. Under the fluorescent lights of commerce, we need to produce *every* day of *every* month of *every* year. Now many of us are beginning to ask, "For what?" As the external world becomes more insecure and even our own bodies become less reliable, we need to access the stability within ourselves that a connection between our body, mind, and spirit would provide.

Some women think they are in contact with their bodies because they take care of them as they would a fine car—they feed them right, exercise them regularly, get them checked over, and take pride in their accomplishments and appearance. But this is done with a sense of separation, even of ownership. The mind, the smart part, is taking care of the body, the dumb part, that they need to carry them around. Whether they do it from vanity or good sense, the caring does not come from within the body's own wisdom.

From the outside, from the mind and the will, we impose diets and exercise that are foreign to the body's true needs. This is from the belief that I *own* my body. This is treating our bodies as objects or possessions. The unspoken agreement is: I will take good care of it and it will work for me. When that agreement is violated by accident or illness, we are often outraged and deeply frightened.

Our first signs of aging are equally disillusioning. We can't trade our body in for a new model at the first dent or sign of shabbiness. Coming home to our body means to understand that we *are* our body, that body wisdom is far deeper and wiser than the intellectual mind, and that we need our body's connection to the larger Universe of which we are a part.

It is also time now for us to become aware of the dance of energy running through our bodies in every moment. Our bodies are actually the densest part of this energy, but we extend out far beyond the body. When we are asleep to the ebbs and flows of our own energy fields, we have little regard for the rhythms of our lives. We dance to the rhythm of the timeclock instead of to the music of our own energy.

We are equally out of touch with our kinesthetic senses— the sense of pleasure and comfort we get from touch. Touch has become isolated and sexualized. It has become suspect.

Coming home to our body means to understand that we *are* our body, that body wisdom is far deeper and wiser than the intellectual mind …

Women need to get back in touch with sensory pleasure from within their own bodies so they can feel the flow of life from a centered place in their own belly. The bookstores are full of books on how to please a man and sexual manuals of all kinds. We need to discover how to please *ourselves* so that self-loving, creative, sensual energy flows unblocked within us.

This book can teach you how to begin to know your body/mind so that you can no longer speak of it as two separate parts of your beingness, how to be awake to the first sign of stress or discomfort so that changes can be made before disease becomes a reality in your life. Dis-ease is exactly what it says, lack of comfort in your body/mind. Many women I meet are so far out of touch with themselves that they no longer have any clear idea of what comfort or pleasure is, except in terms of the addictions that give us pleasure by numbing us to our discomfort.

We are an addictive society precisely because we have lost our way on the road that leads us home to our own body wisdom. In this book I hope to teach you step by step to walk that road again to wholeness, so that when someone asks you how you *feel* about something, you can check inside and answer from the part of your body/mind that knows. This is a totally different experience than answering from the intellect. As one of my first teachers, Brugh Joy, used to say, "The mind is the last to know anything."

The sixties and seventies brought a wake-up call to women in this culture. We woke up to the facts of our oppression from without, from the male-dominated social system. We woke up on that level and marched out to liberate ourselves with creative work. Now we can all hear the clear sound of another wake-up call spreading throughout the land, wherever women talk to women. Let's wake up to the realization that our lives are out of balance, that peace of mind, comfort in the body, and connection with our own spirit are not found outside of ourselves. We must now look *within* in ways that are natural to the feminine and find integration.

Chapter One

HOW TO USE THIS BOOK

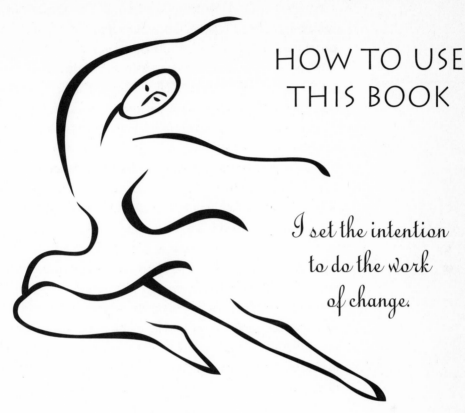

*I set the intention
to do the work
of change.*

For years I was unconsciously searching for the perfect female role model. Every time I read about mentors and role models I wanted one of my own, someone who would lead me forward on my life path, show me the way, teach me the steps, and be my loving guide. Like many women of my generation, mine was a solitary path of growth. I felt alone and different much of the time, so I kept my antennae out for potential guides wherever I went. I would meet or read of different women whom I admired greatly in certain areas, but in other areas of their lives I would not want to be like them at all. I never found one woman that I wanted to emulate.

Finally I realized that the ideal I was looking for doesn't exist, and indeed could not exist. She represents the ideal built into my own psyche, my picture of my Higher Self, a product of my own particular history and values. I worked on developing a clear picture of that ideal woman I wanted to become, made up of all of the qualities I admire. Each one of us will have a different image that completely reflects our own inner feminine.

Here is *my* ideal of a powerful woman—she radiates peace and has a deep inner calm, yet can act decisively whenever necessary; she takes life's events in stride, responding with a sense of humor to all the blocks in her path; she can reach out to others and to life with love and passion, yet also honor her own need to have time alone; she makes choices from her own inner wisdom and creativity, and not from the tugging and pulling of other's needs or the needs of her own inner child.

I now keep this vision of wholeness in the background of my awareness as I move along my life path. I accept who I am in *this* moment, while knowing in my deepest inner wisdom that whatever life struggles I work through will bring me closer to my goal. I consider myself a work of art in progress. Sometimes I find I am sprinting along my path without a moment's hesitation, and other times I wander far afield, feeling lost and small; but my connection with my own body wisdom has become my true guide. It is only because I know how to come home to my body, blending body, mind, and spirit in harmony, that I can even dream of reaching my goal.

It is only
because I know
how to
come home
to my body,
blending
body, mind,
and spirit
in harmony,
that I can even
dream
of reaching
my goal.

Come Home to Your Body

What does it mean to "come home to your body?" Remember a bad day you had recently when you hit the ground running and never did catch up. Everything you did was done in haste and didn't work out as you would have wished. You were crabby and tense, or you played out the martyr or victim role. That was a day run by your mind. You probably didn't check in with your body at all until some part of it hurt. It is probable that you were in some pain by the end of the day because no one was home taking care of your body. These are the days when accidents happen. We don't cut ourselves, fall down, or walk into fixed objects on days when we are centered in our bodies.

Now remember a good day. It probably involved a slower pace or a sense of connectedness in your belly. You were moving from your center and you had time to laugh or talk with someone you love, or touch and be touched. You felt more like reaching out and you could use your senses for pleasure, looking at people and finding them beautiful, smelling fresh air or hearing musical sounds, tasting rich and subtle flavors. All the necessary things got done effortlessly and you chose to be at peace with what did not get done. You were not tormented by impossible lists and perfectionist standards. This was a day of being more at home in your body. It could be called living from a heart-centered place.

We often can't change the external events in our lives. We have only limited power over others. People in your life will be the way they are and will do what is right for them. What we *can* change is our reaction to people and events, and we can bring the awareness of being centered in our body into even our craziest days.

That is what I hope to teach you in this book. I am sure you have heard a million times that the secret to happiness is to be in the NOW moment. Stop having and doing, and become a human *being*. What I have found with many of the women I have worked with over the years is that they don't have any idea how to go about the process of *being*, so they have no choice. By using the simple tools in this book, you will eventually learn to use your body comfort as a constant guide in your life. You will be clear immediately when you have lost touch with your body, just as you would notice it right now if you stopped breathing or if your heart stopped beating.

The three symbols in the margin will remind you to stop and actually do the work as you read.

This symbol means to do the exercise described in the text. Stretch your body/mind a little, make a leap and embody this new learning.

This symbol means to think or remember. My stories are in the book in order to evoke your own stories, your own life experiences.

This symbol reminds you to use your notebook to record your thoughts, feelings, and experiences. You will also see it where I have recommended other books to read about the chapter subject.

Reading about concepts and ideas can evoke some productive inner dialog, but when you feel an experience in your own body/mind, then the new learning is yours forever.

My Own Journey

I want to begin by telling you a part of my own journey so you can appreciate the path that has led to the writing of this book. During the seventies I was a supermom with a business of my own. I had six employees, I had an organic garden, I kept bees and chickens, and I remodeled the house in my spare time. I was a crazy woman. I worked all the time and I had ideas for more work streaming through my brain constantly. I was a successful, creative dynamo and didn't even realize how completely out of balance I was. My personal relationships were a disaster because I didn't understand why everyone didn't want to work as hard as I did. I was driven.

Someone I respected told me I needed to take a yoga class. I loved it passionately and the practice changed my life. Yoga started me on the path toward wholeness. After a few years of dedicated practice of asanas and meditation, I was much more in touch with my body and I had wonderful mystical experiences. Then I gradually came to realize that the underlying belief of this form of yoga was that the spiritual life was all-important and the body was just a temple to house the soul. There was a denial of the vitality of the emotions and the power of the creative force of sexuality.

I started studying psychology and moved on to transformational psychology and energy work with Brugh Joy and Carolyn Conger. Once again I loved it. It made such sense. I learned about the energy fields of the body, how to heal with energy, how to feel the energy fields of others. I was fascinated, but I was still outside my body looking in—this time from another system, another level of awareness.

Of course, at the time, I couldn't articulate my search clearly to myself. I really had no idea what I was looking for. I just knew, once again, that I hadn't quite found it yet. Mystics say we all have a divine spark of unrest within us that drives us on to be the best we can be. I believe that. Never underestimate the power of this divine discontent within you. If you listen to this force it will lead you on, step by step, toward the perfection of your beingness.

Never underestimate the power of this divine discontent within you.

Bodywork

Next I tried learning various forms of bodywork—Trager and massage. I wanted to be a healer and heal with my hands. I had been healing with energy for some time, but for many people this kind of healing was too esoteric and unstructured, even unbelievable. They could not *feel* the energy flow in their bodies. It has been fewer than two hundred years since allopathic medicine discovered the flow of blood throughout the body.

Before then no one believed in, or felt the flow of, their own blood. The time will soon come when people will check their own energy pulsation throughout the day, as we now check our pulse while exercising.

At that time, the tools of Trager bodywork and massage were understandable to more people. I felt I was getting closer to my goal. The problem this time was that people would come to me from their crazy lives, lie down on the table, and let me fix them. They got up feeling wonderful and went back to their craziness. Since they didn't participate in any way in their own healing, they didn't stay fixed. The next week they were back again. I began to feel like a medic on the battlefield. Suddenly that story about giving a hungry woman a fish and she is fed for a day, but teach her how to fish and you have fed her for a lifetime, started to make really good sense to me. I took some time out while I consumed everything I could find about every kind of alternative healing.

The Feldenkrais Method®

Then I discovered the Feldenkrais Method®. Named after the Israeli scientist who developed it, it is a method of teaching the brain by moving the body. By making very small and sometimes unusual movements, we can release blocks and pain in the body and learn new, more useful ways of interacting with our environment. The key is awareness. When you know what you are doing, you can do what you want; until then you are a puppet.

The work is about learning new choices, and it demands the interaction of the practitioner, as teacher, and the student. The Feldenkrais student has a completely different responsibility than the client of a healer. This student knows she is going to have to do the major part of the work of change. To me this was a big step in the right direction. I joined a training group and over a four-year period rolled around on the floor for hours making odd and wonderful movements. I connected with my body in the way I had been seeking for years. It was magical.

Moshe Feldenkrais had two criteria for health: the ability to recover from shock and the ability to live out one's avowed dreams. Can you sense how large that definition is and how few people in this world are achieving it? Stop and think about it for a moment. A paralyzed person like Stephen Hawking, the brilliant physicist, is living out his dream of understanding the world in a new way, and so would be considered healthy by Moshe.

Feldenkrais had a very scientific mind. He thought energy work was New Age and therefore highly suspect, but since I already had that knowledge in my repertoire, this was the final link. I was home. Gradually, in my practice of teaching rather than healing, I discovered and clarified my life purpose. I realized that the keys to my growth have been to listen to my inner wisdom and to trust my body, being willing to be present with it. When I am in this space I am completely aligned on my life path.

My mission is to teach other women how to contact *their* inner wisdom and connect with *their* bodies in a profound and lasting way, so that they can each find their own particular life path. We are all so miraculously unique and we each have our own life purpose, and yet we can all use the same simple tools of self-awareness to guide us. We are all headed in the same direction, toward the union of body, mind, and Spirit.

> We are all so miraculously unique and we each have our own life purpose, and yet we can all use the same simple tools of self-awareness to guide us.

Opening to Spirit

Now, to begin at the beginning, I want to guide you step by step into being in the NOW moment. In this moment, what counts is being at home in your body, content and feeling connected with the rest of the Universe. You may have a chronic condition of dis-ease, such as arthritis, manifesting in your body, but that does not automatically prevent you from experiencing contentment. We all know people who are suffering from terrible physical ailments who are totally open and heart-centered, while others with the very same affliction are acting out the victim pattern. It doesn't matter what our particular life drama is about. It *is* possible to be in a state of inner peace and connection with both our body and our Spirit.

When I speak of Spirit I am speaking of the life force that runs through us but is much bigger than us, that connects us to the mystery of source and to the larger dimensions of life. When we open to the part of us that is Spirit, we can see our life lessons more clearly and move out of the "Why me?" space into a larger perspective.

I was hesitant to mention the word Spirit in my work for many years. For some people it has a religious connotation and they immediately back away. Gradually, I found that if I don't anchor my teaching and my healing to the larger dimension of who we are and what we are doing in *this* body, at *this* time, the lessons don't stay learned. Our daily dramas are such a small, though compelling, part of who we are. The deeper parts of us, our Inner Wisdom and our Higher Self, are always waiting patiently for us to remember that.

Workbook Suggestions

Here are my recommendations for how to get the most out of this book. This is a WORKbook, so if you skip the exercises, it won't work for you. I have a friend who buys all the "right" books but never makes time to read them or do the work involved. We joke that she has the most evolved bookshelf on this planet.

 ✳   Get a notebook and write down all that you notice as you work your way through the book. Writing is an interesting thing; some people love it and some people hate it. Anything we learned to do in school seems to evoke automatic resistance in some of us. This writing is for you alone. Don't bother with grammar or spelling or punctuation. Just put your pen to the paper and let your words spill out as if you were talking to yourself. If you get stuck, write the words "I am" or "I feel" and see what follows. You don't have to do it any certain way. Just write.

When I go over and over in my head about a problem, I never seem to be able to resolve it. The very act of writing it down always brings me more clarity. Also, my insights are right there in black and white if I get pulled into the same pattern again. It is amazing how repetitive our life dramas are and we often don't realize it until we write them down. There are some wonderful books on writing that I will include in the resource list at the end of this chapter, but for now all you need to do is start. In some sense, I always find that writing clears my slate and lets me start again, fresh and new and open.

✳ Complete the chapters in order, one a week if possible. If you need more time then take it, but not so long that you lose momentum. If you are a person who learns slowly, then do one chapter a month. By having a planned time period, you avoid drifting away from your purpose. If you hate or resist any particular chapter, notice that reaction. It's always very interesting to note what we resist; often it is the very thing we need to do the most, but give yourself permission to skip it and take what you need. You may choose to come back to it later. If you were my client, I would tailor the experience just for you.

Resistance is a key to discomfort and I always check inside myself to see where my resistance is coming from. Sometimes it comes from the part of me that is resistant to any change at all or any work at all; even so, we don't learn well under coercion. We all have different ways that are comfortable for us to learn new skills. I have tried to incorporate many choices. If you are a predominantly aural person, put some of the exercises on tape and listen to them. My chief bias is that the best way for anyone to learn is by personal experience. Sometimes we can remember experiences we have already had and look at them in a new way.

✳ Each chapter begins with an affirmation. Write it out, big and in color, and stick it on your bathroom mirror and refrigerator door. Allow it to dance around in the back of your mind every day and say it before you go to sleep. Affirmations are a great way to utilize the enormous power of the mind. I don't ever intend to belittle that power when I push for more equality for body and Spirit.

✳ If you could inspire a group of three or four women to work with you and meet once a week to share, it would be enormously helpful. We are all different and we are all alike. A support group can clarify things for you and save you time and pain. Ask around but don't over-persuade. People who are pushed into it won't go the distance, and that could affect your determination. Women really supporting women in their growth is one of the most wonderful experiences we can share.

Moving into the world of business has caused many women to become competitive, but that is not our nature. We are cooperative beings and we have been isolated for far too long. I am in several women's groups of various kinds right now and I am always amazed at how much we all learn from each others' experience. We don't have to re-invent the wheel. By resonating with another woman's experience we can see our own life stories in a new way. The love and support and honest feedback I get from my groups has accelerated my growth and deeply enriched my life. I am enormously grateful for them.

✳ Make a commitment to yourself to work through the whole book no matter what comes up in your life to interfere. The tools are designed to be done mostly during your normal life. They won't take an enormous amount of extra time from your schedule. On the few occasions when they do, you are worth it.

✳   Be curious. Curiosity is vital to an interesting life. Remember how babies are endlessly curious. They play with their fingers and toes for hours. They try new things a trillion times before settling on the best way for them. If we had all given up at the third or fourth try, we would still be lying on our backs like beached turtles. You now become the object of your own curiosity. YOU are fascinating. How do you act? How do you move? What makes you feel good or bad? What reaction does a certain external event have on your physical body?

This isn't a scientific method. We will never get consensus and absolutely nothing is repeatable in exactly the same way. We are all unique at each unique moment in time. That alone is such a miracle. A client told me last week that she was not open to feeling energy move through her because it wasn't scientific. "It's just anecdotal," she said with scorn. Learn to *trust* your own experiences. Don't take my word for anything. Don't give up too soon, and don't close your mind to new possibilities.

I rarely use statistics or quotes or footnotes because I don't believe in them. Statistics and studies can be quoted to prove anything, and also the opposite. I will include some books in the resource lists at the end of each chapter that are full of amazing statistics and studies about the body/mind connection, but for now I want you to have the direct experience of each lesson. Remember that when you feel it in your own body, it is yours forever.

Remember that when you feel it in your own body, it is yours forever.

Changing From the Inside

You will probably find that some chapters remind you of things you have done in the past or have heard a hundred times before, while some ideas may be completely new to you. See if you can move to "beginner's mind" with each exercise and do it as if it were the first time you have ever seen it. There is always a way to deepen our experience if we don't assume we already know all there is to know about a subject. Rather than thinking of the lessons of life as a ladder on which the tests become progressively harder as we move up (which is a left-brain concept), try to think of them as unfolding in layers, like the layers of an onion or the petals of a lotus, to reveal a new richness at each depth.

I have tried to keep both the information and the lessons as simple and direct as possible. Watching women among men, I am always struck by the sophistication of our language and the intellectual discussion of concepts and ideas, often with the swirling undercurrent of competition for attention. In groups of women, in a nonbusiness setting, the language becomes simpler and more honest, sharing from the heart and from our emotions. We may cry, but we always laugh a lot. We love to tell our stories, the small vignettes of our lives that reveal us completely. It is this level I am trying to evoke in you. I ask simple questions so that you can look inside and rediscover your own history, your own mythology.

Your own body wisdom knows what you need to do to be happy and at peace with the world.

This book is not going to fix your relationships or make you thin. If you have no money or a job you hate or a life-threatening disease, this book can't fix those things. What it can do is change your life from the inside, as you live from a more integrated place. When your body, mind, and Spirit are in alignment, you have access to all the answers you need about healing the particular pains and lacks in your life. Your own body wisdom knows what you need to do to be happy and at peace with the world. We just can't hear the message over the constant chatter in our heads and in our lives.

One of my clients, Evalynn, said that as she watched her mother in her eighties become more and more infirm, she was deeply afraid that she was following along on the same downward path. For her, this was a wake-up call. She woke up to her disconnection from her body. After doing the lessons in this book, and some other Feldenkrais work, she had renewed hope in her own ability to create a healthy future. We have enough ninety-year-old women as role models who are bursting with energy and health and still enjoying life to know that we have that choice, if we commit to taking care of our body/minds from this moment forward.

A special note: If you have a history of physical or sexual abuse, it may be more difficult for you to use some of the tools in this book. I have worked with many women with horrendous histories, and eventually, they learned to be present in their bodies, so I am convinced it can be done. A child dealing with pain that is not understandable or bearable will learn to leave her body. This is the only way our body wisdom can protect us. It even happens to adults.

If we can't fight and we can't run, we freeze. When we freeze, we leave our bodies and go somewhere in our minds where pain and betrayal can't reach us. One client used to count the threads in the chenille bedspread, another could reproduce the pattern of the wallpaper in the room she had when she was four. We may fear coming back to full aliveness from that time on, so we watch our lives from a distance. A vital trust in our own body has been violated. So, although some of what you read here may seem to be impossible or unreal or just not applicable to you, please bear with it. If you can't do something in the exercises, then first imagine yourself doing it. The blocks will soften with self-loving repetition.

Once you feel, even in a small way, the joy of being present in this moment, then your trust in your own body will grow. Trusting can be re-learned even when we had good reason to reject it. When you are finally in your own body as an adult woman, when you listen to it carefully and heed its warnings, it will keep you safe.

Resource List

Rico, Gabriele Lusser. *Writing the Natural Way.* Los Angeles: J. P. Tarcher, Inc., 1983.

Goldberg, Natalie. *Writing Down the Bones.* Boston: Shambhala Publishing, 1986.

Chopra, Deepak. *Quantum Healing.* New York: Bantam Books, 1990.

Chapter Two

TOOLS OF AWARENESS

*With awareness
I am present
in each moment.*

ost of the lessons in this book will work on awakening your self-awareness. In the normal sequence of learning, once an action or behavior is
learned, it becomes more automatic and requires less attention. In this
way, most actions and thoughts in our daily lives become habitual and move outside
of our conscious awareness; our body sensations, in particular, sink below the threshold of our conscious mind. We have all had the experience of walking or driving
somewhere, deep in thought, and arriving without really knowing how we got there.
Another common experience is to walk past someone we know without seeing them.
We seem to be on automatic pilot during much of our daily lives.

15

This unconscious repetition of our habitual patterns is often very useful to us. If we tried to become conscious of every repetitive act we do in just one day we would go crazy, but without awareness there is no possibility of change. What we are going to practice this week is a special kind of selective awareness. For example, right now you are reading this book; your attention is focused on the written words. Now add to your awareness the body sensations of sitting, but without changing your sitting posture in any way. It's almost impossible, isn't it? The act of noticing *itself* will subtly change anything.

Try again. Notice your breathing. Is it high in your chest or deep in your belly? Are you hunched over in any way so that you have difficulty taking a full breath? As you thought about it, did you straighten up? Notice the place on your spine between your shoulder blades. Are you holding tension there? Notice your shoulders. Are they up around your ears? Did you change them if they were? Were you able to read this passage and notice your body sensations at the same time? In general, women have the ability to utilize multiple awareness because this is a function of the right side of the brain. Most of us can easily prepare a meal, listen to a conversation, and keep one eye on children playing, all at the same time.

Refining your ability to tune into your body sensations while you continue with your normal life will probably be relatively easy for you. The *value* in learning to include these sensations in your awareness lies in your ability to prevent chronic pain from becoming part of your reality. *Chronic* means pain that is long-standing, recurs again and again, or is always there but in varying degrees. Pain is a message from our body, and becomes chronic only when the message has been ignored for too long. Most pain, from accidents on the job to carpal tunnel syndrome to migraines, can be prevented long before it occurs by staying in constant touch with the comfort level of your body. Pain is *not* a necessary part of the aging process.

Noticing

The primary tool of awareness is the habit of noticing. It's almost instantaneous, almost effortless, and yet can relieve your body of many of the stresses and strains of your daily life. Women customarily carry their stress in their shoulders. When do *you* normally pay attention to the tension in your shoulders? Is it after you get home from work, or just before bed as you finally let go of the day? Or is it only when the sensation becomes very painful? We have so many claims on our attention that it seems the claim of our body sensation is most often ignored.

Some years ago I had a stressful job and a long drive home. About thirty minutes after I left work, still thinking about my day, I would drive through a tunnel. Perhaps because of the darkness of the tunnel, I would suddenly notice my shoulders up next to my ears and consciously let them down with a sigh of relief. I got in the habit of using the tunnel as a signal to change from my working self to my evening self, leaving my job concerns behind and letting go of the tension in my shoulders.

The trick to noticing is the curiosity I mentioned earlier. If it's just another thing to remember to do in your day, you will probably resist it. Try thinking of noticing as a positive, interesting way to use your mind when you would otherwise be worrying about your problems. Instead of rerunning, for the hundredth time, the argument you are having with the imaginary person in your head, watch what your body is doing. That is one of the main differences between humans and animals. A cat is prepared in an instant to fight or flee danger, and when the danger is past, she doesn't sit and agonize about it, she gets back to full relaxation. We have such big, advanced brains that we get to replay our worst moments again and again.

Imagine that human beings and their behavior are one of the most intriguing and entertaining puzzles in the world. Have you ever caught yourself behaving in some way (yelling or nagging or flirting, for instance) and wondered who on earth got inside you? It is fascinating to watch ourselves use our bodies to interact with each other. Notice the changes in your body posture when someone you are attracted to, or want to impress, approaches you. Learning to consciously read body language, both our own and others, is so useful. We all read each other all the time on an intuitive level already; bringing that skill into conscious awareness will benefit you enormously. When you start noticing your own behaviors through your body movements, you will start on a voyage of discovery that can last your whole life long.

One large problem with developing the habit of noticing is our old habit of self-judgment. Be aware that we all have an inner critic, a part of our subconscious mind that we created as a child. It is usually our internalized parent, so it can operate as either a loving guide or, most often, a harsh detractor. Since many of our parents were pretty unconscious about childrearing, it is usually safe to assume that your inner critic is often too picky and downright rude for your peace of mind. In fact, the inner critic is probably one of the reasons we went unconscious in the first place. So be very sure that you don't use noticing for extra ammunition to criticize yourself. There is no right or wrong here; you can leave out judgment entirely. This is not another opportunity to make yourself feel bad.

Go back to the time before you judged yourself as right or wrong, as a failure or a success. That would be a very young age for most of us. Our inner critic is born very early and gathers enormous power. Notice your feelings and actions now with the joyful spirit of curiosity and exploration.

Here is a simple example of this technique: I can notice that I habitually sit with my whole spine leaning on one elbow as I work at my desk. I now have choices:

✳   I can continue as I am.

✳   I can move to a more balanced position so I don't increase the tension in my shoulders and spine.

✳ I can nag at myself for sitting so poorly. Most of us have the "sit up straight" voice of our parents and early teachers deeply embedded in our bodies and minds.

If I notice that I often nag myself, this is valuable information. The inner critic often nags away at you in the background of your thoughts, taking the shine off your self-esteem without your conscious attention. I may choose to change this pattern of automatic self-blame in order to make my life more comfortable. It is possible to put your inner critic on reduced duty, a kind of semi-retired status. The first step toward doing that is to notice it.

If I utilize the second choice of adjusting my sitting posture into balance, then I could prevent future misalignment and probable pain. If I decide to keep on sitting and leaning, I am now doing it consciously. Whatever choice I make, I am winning; noticing—bringing some act or behavior into the light of conscious awareness—is a winning strategy.

Noticing Effort

The first thing I have my clients notice is the amount of extra effort they put into their daily tasks. Many of them have said that this awareness alone started a process of change that led to great transformation.

Cathy, a client, was completely unaware of the level of tension she always held in her body. Her movements were jerky and stiff. She wondered why her muscles were always in knots and also why no one seemed comfortable when she was around. She said she would love to be relaxed and peaceful but she wasn't that kind of person and never had been. She lived alone and didn't really trust people to like her, so she had a hard time making friends. She started noticing small things about the effort she made in her movements and she said, "It is almost as if I am fighting with myself, deep down inside, about every movement I make. I think people are watching me when they aren't. When I do everything more gently, with less effort, the world seems to shift into another focus. I see things differently." Before long she was able to move out of her mind, back inside her body, and her life really did transform.

How much effort do you put into doing your daily repetitive tasks, all the things you do mindlessly every day?

✻   Notice how tightly you hold your hairbrush or your toothbrush.

✻   How firmly do you clasp your fork while eating or your knife while cutting?

✻   How firmly or gently do you place something on the table?

✻   How hard do your feet hit the ground?

✻   Do you frown or make faces as you think?

✻   How firmly do you hold the telephone to your ear?

✻   How aggressive are your gestures?

✻   How loud is your voice?

✻   Are your movements jerky or smooth?

✻   Are you usually in a hurry?

Many of us wear out our joints with extra effort, in the same way that jogging on concrete will wear out your knee and hip joints faster than walking on grass. The joints in our hands, wrists, and shoulders especially show the effects of a lifetime of holding on too tight.

The amount of effort we use also gives us clues to our emotional state. When we are peaceful and loving, our movements will tend to be smoother and softer. I always knew when my mother was upset by the way she brushed my hair. My parents never argued in front of us, but some days I wished I were bald and I thought I probably soon would be. My mother would tug and jerk and pull on my frizzy, permed curls until my whining brought her back to attention. She laughs about it now that she is a laid back Californian, but the other women she worked with used to say, "Just get Joan mad and she'll work like ten men." Since her life was often frustrating, the floors were always polished, the brass gleamed, and the windows shone. It was unexpressed anger translating into effort.

During the learning phase of acquiring a new skill, it is normal to use more effort and involve more muscles than we need. We have all seen people with their faces scrunched up, learning how to write or draw. It doesn't help, actually. While learning to ride a bicycle, you can probably remember the fear that kept many of your muscles tight and tense and made it much harder for you to learn. Gradually, with practice, we move into the area of competence and start to relax all the muscles not necessary to completing the task.

Most of us stop at the level of competence and never go any further. In the case of biking, our bike is a tool to get us where we need to go. There are some people, however, who will fall in love with biking and they will move beyond competence into the level of the lyrical, where they and their bike become one. To watch their effortless movement is a joy. They are in the flow space. Is there anything that *you* do so well that you become lyrical and flowing and forget effort?

While noticing effort, you may also make the discovery that you don't put *enough* effort into what you do. Most women work too hard for their own good (a historical pattern), but there is an opposite pattern of insecurity that some of us show the world. Then we are so tentative, so soft, so gentle, that we seem ineffective at everything we do. We whisper when we talk, ask permission for everything, and apologize constantly. If you think this applies to you, even in one or two of your life roles, you could practice turning up the effort bit by bit until you get the respect every woman deserves. None of us has to apologize for being present. We all have our own unique collection of skills and talents, and we have as much right to be here as the next person.

Spend the first two days of this week noticing the amount of effort you use without trying to change it. Notice also what frame of mind or emotion seems to accompany excessive effort. The next two days, experiment with varying your effort and finding out the minimum amount it takes to complete a task efficiently. Notice if decreasing the work involved in many of your daily routine tasks makes an appreciable difference in your life. For many of my clients, just this small change is the beginning of the wake-up process.

Try an Experiment

Sit comfortably at a desk or table and pick up an object like a plastic or metal cup. Holding it as tight as possible, bang it down on the table forcefully. Allow your attention to travel through your body while you are doing this until you are clear which muscles are tight and involved in this action, and which are not. Do you notice anything happening in your jaw or your face? How about your thighs and buttocks? Are you feeling any emotion? Now gradually ease off the force and effort, repeating the same movement more softly and gently. What changes? Are fewer muscles involved?

Now put the cup down as silently and gently as possible and notice if the tension returns when you are trying too hard to achieve gentleness. At what point does the softness turn into an *effort* to be soft? In the same way, it takes more effort to shout or to whisper than it does to talk within a normal range.

Now think of the words *grace* and *elegance* and pick up and put down the cup with those qualities in your awareness. Did the quality of your movement change again? Isn't grace the very absence of effort, the smooth flow of natural movement? The ideal movement is one that uses all the muscles that need to be used for accomplishment and no more.

Grimacing or scowling as we write, or tightening our shoulders as we think, is called "parasitic movement." It is unnecessary action. Can you imagine the amount of energy you would have left over at the end of the day if you always moved with grace, involving all the necessary muscles and the necessary effort and no more?

Most of the women I have worked with do not believe themselves to be graceful. Maybe it is a skewed sample since they are all seeking help with movement or pain, but even the professional dancers I know often have the same belief. Moshe Feldenkrais said that in movement we can make the impossible possible, the possible effortless, and the effortless elegant. But you can't achieve elegance and grace from the outside—from the mind. Your awareness has to be *inside* the body, and then elegance is effortless.

Many of us checked out of our bodies when we hit the gawky, clumsy stage at puberty—when we were embarrassed about our growth and bewildered by our hormonal changes. We confused our appearance with our essence, and a pimple became a tragedy. Start checking back in to your body on a regular basis. Pick one small movement you do often, like picking up your coffee cup, and make it smoother and more flowing. It isn't so very difficult to make our small everyday movements graceful? Experiment. Don't make hard work of it. You could be the first woman to make drinking coffee a lyrical experience.

Doing It to the Max

Begin to notice the times when you do movements "to the maximum," even though going halfway would be enough. This is slightly different than over-efforting.

Try this: Stand up and raise your left arm to the ceiling. Try hard; do it to the maximum. What did you learn? Now raise your arm very slowly and feel *how* you do it. Which part of you starts the motion, then what muscles kick in? When does your shoulder get involved? What are your eyes doing? Are you making faces? What are your feet doing to participate? Don't

It is
wonderful
and productive
to have goals,
but if we can't
be present
during the
process of
reaching them,
then we have
bypassed
most of our
lives.

stretch as far as you could. Instead of being goal-oriented, be process-oriented. It's a whole different experience.

It is wonderful and productive to have goals, but if we can't be present during the process of reaching them, then we have bypassed most of our lives. After all, when you achieve a goal, what happens? You usually start out immediately toward another one. You may as well enjoy the journey.

Our culture encourages the habit of trying hard and doing everything to the maximum—it's part of our socialization. Do your best. Strive for perfection. If at first you don't succeed, try, try, try again. This frantic striving can wear us out before our time because it doesn't take into account the ebbs and flows of life. Doing dishes isn't the same as doing micro-surgery. Sometimes we can just settle back and coast. We can get by on less effort and stop wearing ourselves out with such high expectations. Then when it comes to the goals or tasks we care about deeply, we can use the extra energy we have to do our very best.

I've already admitted that I used to be a compulsive worka-holic, and on some days I put out maximum effort at maxi-mum speed for sixteen to eighteen hours. I would crawl into bed still feeling as if I had not accomplished enough. If only there were more hours in the day, I could have done it all!

Then a young woman came to work for me, and when I was obsessing about doing something perfectly she would say, "Pam, this is not brain surgery, is it? What will this mat-ter in a hundred years?" At first I was totally shocked. Her attitude was completely foreign to me, but gradually it start-ed to make sense. Now she is a dear friend and our favorite saying is "Life is too short." It's too short to spend in anything less than peace and happiness, with some passion thrown in. Don't wear yourself out on the small stuff. You wouldn't dream of cooking all your meals at 550 degrees. Back off on your own energy use; your body will last longer and you'll enjoy it more.

Questioning Your Observations

After noticing your behavior for a while, you may find that you ask yourself questions about it. In this context, behavior means a group of movements that you make. Riding a bicycle is a behavior that has many movements in common for all of us. Getting upset is a behavior that may have extremely diverse movements for different people. For one person, getting upset may involve running away and crying. For another, it may involve shaking her fists, thrusting out her chin, and yelling. Another woman may make microscopic movements of her lower lip and eyelids and tighten the rest of her body until it is numb and silent. *All* of these reactions could be produced by the same external event. We are all different and we are all the product of our own particular history. I love the saying, "Our bodies are the shapes of the joys and sorrows that have formed us" because it is so true.

We usually have patterns of behavior that echo those of our parents (or oppose them). When I was in my thirties, I was very aggravated to realize that my mother was living inside me and creating some of my behaviors. For example, I grew up in England where the weather was unpredictable at best. When the sun came out my mother would invariably say, "Go outside and play. It's a shame to be inside on such a beautiful day." Now I live in California; the sun is shining more often than not, and I noticed this strange, uneasy feeling whenever I had to spend the whole day inside. I would feel almost guilty.

The funny part was that Mother also gave me a very strong message about doing something useful with my time, and the importance of being productive. Soon after I moved to California, I developed a passionate interest in gardening and I would work in the garden for hours. I was fulfilling both criteria; I was outside in the sunshine and also working hard and accomplishing something. Since I learned that it was my mother's voice prompting my behavior, I have more choices. I can be less compulsive about gardening, and I can stay inside and work when it is sunny without feeling bad and guilty. It was by asking myself questions that I discovered the root of this behavior.

Some useful questions are:

* How do I do this behavior?

* When do I do this behavior?

* What triggers this behavior?

* Who triggers this behavior?

* Was this behavior learned from one of my parents?

* Do I want to keep on doing this behavior?

The question we normally ask the most, the "Why" question, is much less useful. It comes from linear, logical, cause-and-effect thinking that usually leads to judgment and blame.

For example, I could notice that I feel tightness in my stomach and I have an intense urge to move my legs. These are body sensations that correspond to the "I've got to get out of here" feeling.

I can ask myself the "How" question. First I have increased acid in my stomach, then I tighten up my muscles there and my throat feels tight. Then my buttocks tighten, my knees bend, my legs get restless, and I need to move away.

Then I ask the "When" question. I behave in this way when someone is saying things I don't want to hear, pummeling me with words and not giving me a chance to answer. This also explains what triggers my behavior.

The "Who triggers it" question is, of course, the person I am with right now, but I could also go back in time and remember who originally triggered this behavior. This complex pattern didn't leap fully formed into my life this very instant. Having been brought up in England, where children were not allowed to answer back to adults, I have a whole cast of original triggers, the members too numerous for individual credit.

"Was this behavior learned from one of my parents?" Yes, my mother had the same reaction to confrontation. She would leave the scene.

"Do I want to keep it?" No, I am old enough to stand my ground and face anything I have to. If I'm not old enough yet, then it's not going to happen in *this* lifetime.

So now I can notice my behavior and choose instead to stay and face a verbal assault. Over time, this original reactive behavior would gradually die away and be replaced by a more resourceful response. If I had asked the "Why" question first, I might have come up with the same information, but maybe not.

We are all such wonderfully inventive people, geniuses at self-justification. We learn that very young. When a small child who has just spilled her milk for the second time is asked, "Why did you do that?" she doesn't have any idea. She likes the pattern it makes or she likes the attention. Who knows? Pretty soon we develop good, logical, linear answers to the "Why" questions adults are constantly asking us. It becomes a mark of our success in relating to others. It's called self-rationalization or excuse-making.

There are even cultural fads and preferences in our rationalizations. A few years ago in San Francisco, a man on trial for murder claimed that eating junk food had made him kill. His excuse became known as the Twinkie Defense. Can you imagine that defense being very acceptable in the 1930s? However, during the thirties it *was* accepted that a woman would often act erratically and become unstable during menopause. That is not a valid rationalization used by women today.

The fact is that we all have many consistent, repetitive behaviors. If they do not serve to make our life rich and rewarding, we can notice them first and then change them. "Why" questions often lead to rationalization and judgment, and don't help much with the process of change. Many women with years of psychotherapy can tell you exactly why they behave as they do and yet be powerless to change their reactions. It is by replacing a learned body reaction with a new body action that we accomplish change. Movement creates and anchors change.

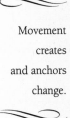

Movement
creates
and anchors
change.

Remembering

Another tool of awareness is remembering, which is actually noticing in the past tense. We have all lived through so much that we can look back on and learn from with the benefit of hindsight. Our perception of past events often changes as the years go by. Do you remember as a teenager not understanding at all why your parents acted the way they did? Then, when you had teenagers of your own, it all became clear to you.

By remembering in full sensory detail, hearing what was said, seeing the whole picture, repeating the body posture, and feeling the feelings we had then, we can use our present level of wisdom and insight to explore our past. We can also see more clearly how our beliefs and opinions were formed. When I ask you to remember something as we travel through the book, stop and give yourself fully to the remembrance, and write in your notebook if you gain new insight. All the women I have known love to tell their own stories. Our stories are valuable: They put our lives into context and help us make sense of our journey. How can we appreciate how far we have come if we never look back to some of the turning points on the way?

Explorations for the Week

✳ Notice the amount of effort you are using.

✳ Decrease the amount of effort necessary to accomplish your tasks.

✳ Introduce a feeling of grace and elegance into your movements.

✳ Notice if you usually do things to the maximum.

✳ If you become aware of an interesting or intriguing behavior, ask yourself the six questions:

How do I do this behavior?

When do I do this behavior?

What triggers this behavior?

Who triggers this behavior?

Was this behavior learned from one of my parents?

Do I want to keep on doing this behavior?

✳ Remember the person in your past who most influenced how hard you work today. Ponder how happy and balanced that person is or was.

Remember to write your insights in your notebook. Let your notebook hold the progress of your changes. Then later, if you feel you aren't accomplishing anything, you can go back and read it and appreciate your growth. We all took a long time to become socialized to the point of working beyond our capacity and tuning out our pain. Let's give ourselves plenty of time for the transformation back into awake and powerful women with body-centered awareness.

Chapter Three

BREATHING

*My breath
connects me with
all life.*

Everyone, without exception, who is reading this book is breathing. Breathing is absolutely vital to us and yet we are usually unconscious of it. It is the *quality* of our breath that determines how alive we are, how awake, how vivacious, even how interesting our life is. Learning to breathe correctly for each situation we are in is the fastest way to change our lives for the better. No matter what emotional or physical pain you are in right now, breathing with awareness will help you to alleviate it. That is a pretty big claim for something so simple to learn, but it is absolutely true.

In my workshops, I often get resistance to breathwork: Breathing is boring; I already know how to breathe; let's do something new and exciting. Trust me.

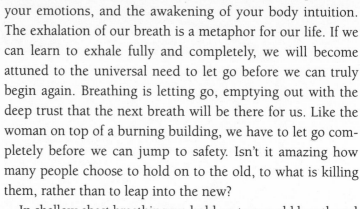

If we can
learn to exhale
fully and
completely,
we will become
attuned to the
universal need
to let go
before we can
truly begin
again.

Breathing is the road home to peace of mind, acceptance of your emotions, and the awakening of your body intuition. The exhalation of our breath is a metaphor for our life. If we can learn to exhale fully and completely, we will become attuned to the universal need to let go before we can truly begin again. Breathing is letting go, emptying out with the deep trust that the next breath will be there for us. Like the woman on top of a burning building, we have to let go completely before we can jump to safety. Isn't it amazing how many people choose to hold on to the old, to what is killing them, rather than to leap into the new?

In shallow chest breathing we hold on to our old breath and never fully exhale. Our blood doesn't get enough oxygen and every cell in our body, especially in the brain, is affected. Deep breathing can slow our brainwaves down to the alpha state. It is only then that we can access our deeper wisdom. Our normal beta brain rhythm is too active to give us time to pay attention to our quiet, powerful voice of inner knowing.

Why do we need to *learn* how to breathe? It is the same old answer. Our lives are out of tune with nature. The socialization process, with all its traumas, robbed us of the space to grow up organically. We learned to hurry up. How many times were you told as a child to hurry up? You limited your full inhalation of the breath of life so that you could keep up with the crazy pace of the adults around you. When you were upset or scared, you held your breath, and you gradually learned that by breathing less deeply you could deaden your feelings. I remember being sad as a child, and lying in bed breathing such small breaths that I imagined I would become invisible and light as a cloud, and I would float away to heaven. It didn't work; I'm still here. If we had been taught as children to breathe *into* our feelings instead of holding our breath in times of trouble, our worlds would be different now. Never mind; it is not too late to learn how to breathe.

The majority of us in the western world breathe into our upper chests most of the time. Look around you. Notice your breath and that of the people you spend time with. Notice how people breathe when they are excited, bored, depressed, rushed, overworked, calm, or loving. If you cannot feel your belly moving in and out against your belt as you breathe, then you are breathing into your upper chest.

Only one half cup of your blood circulates through this upper part of your lungs. Your lungs are designed to oxygenate one quart of blood, so you are asking your body to do the work of energizing and detoxifying your entire system on less than one cup of fuel instead of four. Try making a cake with one egg instead of four and see how flat and dense it becomes. By breathing deeply into your belly, you can function better in this hurry-up world. The paradox is that if we would breathe more deeply, we might have the good sense not to be hurried through our lives. We might slow down to smell the roses and enjoy the pleasures of our senses.

There are special breathing exercises available from many disciplines, and I am going to include here only the three that I like the most and use regularly. This is one of the chapters that requires an investment of time, preferably in the early morning.

Another good time is after work, before you begin your evening activities. If you wait to do the exercise in bed before falling asleep, you may feel calmer, but it is also possible you will feel so full of energy that you may have to get up again. Try it out and find the best timing for yourself. To overcome our unproductive breathing habits, it is important to be regular about this practice.

Rocking Breath

Read through the whole sequence first, then have someone read the instructions to you if possible.

1. Lie on the floor with your knees up and your feet flat. Imagine, as you lie there, that you are a clock on the wall. At your heart is the number twelve and at your knees is the

number six. We will be using this analogy again in a later chapter, so take the time to become familiar with it now. If I were floating on the ceiling above you, looking down, I would see you as a clock face. Your tailbone on the floor is the center of the clock.

2. Now direct your pelvis and belly toward your knees at six o'clock. This is a small movement. Your tailbone does not lift off the floor, but your lower back arches away from the floor and your belly rounds outward. Then rock back and direct your pelvis toward twelve o'clock, at your heart. Your lower back will now press into the floor. Rock gently back and forth between twelve o'clock and six o'clock until you are clear about how this movement feels. Do not work too hard. This is a small and gentle rocking movement. You may know it as the pelvic tilt. You are not pushing with your feet. Your upper back, neck, shoulders, and jaw are fully relaxed.

3. As your belly rounds out toward your knees at six o'clock, inhale a breath deep into your belly. When you are ready to exhale, rock back to twelve o'clock and exhale fully. You are breathing at your own rhythm in an easy, unforced way, and the movement of your pelvis is reminding you of where to breathe in and where to breathe out.

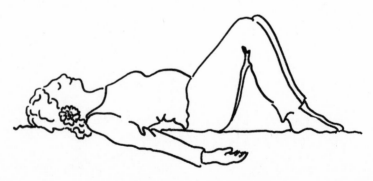

As your belly rounds out, inhale deeply.

Once that is clear, we will work on the exhalation a little more, since it is the exhalation that is the most important part of this breath. The in-breath will always happen automatically if we wait long enough. The out-breath requires work on the part of the diaphragm, the muscular sheet that separates the lungs from the digestive system.

4. Start to exhale through your mouth as if you were blowing out a candle. (The inhalation is still through the nose.) Exhale completely by pulling your diaphragm up under your ribs. See how much more breath you can exhale when your diaphragm is doing its job. Keep your shoulders relaxed and don't tighten your buttocks. Notice all the extra muscles you are tensing because you are learning something new. Let them all go.

5. Each time you are completely empty of air, wait until the in-breath comes by itself, deep into your belly. Decrease the effort and blowing of the out-breath until it is soft and gentle and takes twice as long as the in-breath. You are still rocking to remind you where the breath goes. If you try to breathe in when your back is flat against the floor, you will not be able to breath deeply. Let your belly expand and contract. This movement is good for your stomach muscles.

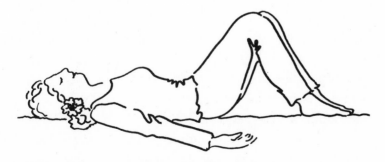

Exhale completely by pulling your diaphragm up under your ribs.

This exercise may sound complicated, but it really isn't. Once you have learned it, practice for five minutes every day to start your day with a sense of balance and personal power. I also recite a mantra in my head on every exhalation. "There is always enough time" is one of my favorites. You can do this breath in bed before you get up, but in the beginning, the hard floor against your backbone makes it easier to learn.

Here is a reminder list:

* Keep your knees up.

* Tilt pelvis toward six o'clock.

* Arch your back as you breathe into your belly.

* Tilt pelvis toward twelve o'clock.

* Press your back into the floor as you breathe out slowly and fully through rounded lips, pulling your diaphragm up under your ribs.

* Wait for new in-breath to come naturally.

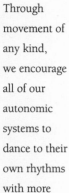

Through movement of any kind, we encourage all of our autonomic systems to dance to their own rhythms with more energy and aliveness.

Some Buddhists believe that the space between the breaths is where enlightenment can occur. That space gets longer with this practice, but it has nothing to do with holding your breath. It is a clear moment of no time when you can feel your heartbeat moving through you.

You may have discovered while practicing this exercise that your diaphragm was completely unknown to you. Many of us have allowed our diaphragm to lie around for years on permanent vacation status. By relearning to involve it in our breathing process, we are also helping our digestion. Every internal event in our body happens to its own rhythm, and by allowing your diaphragm to sit out the dance for so long, other parts of you may have become sluggish also. Through movement of any kind, we encourage all of our autonomic systems— immune, digestive, lymph, endocrine, etc.—to dance to their own rhythms with more energy and aliveness. Can't you just imagine all of these movements inside us, like in a huge dance hall where everyone hears their own music and dances to their own tune. Some are doing a polka, some are doing swing, no one is sitting out. No one is a wallflower.

As you continue to practice this exercise for five minutes a day, you may become more aware of your breathing throughout your day. Whenever you do become aware of your breath, take a few deep belly breaths and exhale fully. Very soon, upper chest breathing will feel restrictive to you and will be a sign of tension that will wake you up to your bodily discomfort.

I want to say something about bellies here. Belly breathing may have been deliberately unlearned by us as young women as soon as we became vain. I cannot deny that breathing into your belly will make your belly move in and out. If it doesn't, you aren't doing it correctly. Look at some old pictures of movie stars from the fifties. They all have nice round bellies— Marilyn Monroe, for example. This is normal and healthy. The body image we have been compressed into since Twiggy was popular is completely unnatural and unhealthy. It's a mental straitjacket as dangerous as a Victorian corset. I am not envious when I see someone with a ladder-muscled stomach. They are restricting their aliveness in a serious way.

During my training, there was a lot of joking about a Feldenkrais belly—a belly that moves with the breath, that can give space for digestion, that is strong enough to help support our spine, but never rigid. I don't understand how the starving orphan look, and the Barbie doll look, ever took such a deep hold on the female psyche. Breathe deeply into your belly and blow that image far out of your life.

The Humming Breath

This second breath can be practiced anytime, anywhere. First try to hum on a shallow chest breath. Then hum a tune without thinking about breathing. You will notice that you naturally take a quick belly breath in order to have enough air to hum properly. During the day, whenever you remember, hum a tune you like. This works especially well when you feel yourself tensing up or reacting to your life in a negative way.

Don't let yourself think of reasons why you can't hum. You aren't trying out for the opera. *Anyone can hum.* It is great for your vocal chords. Allow the sound to drop down from your head to your belly. Hear the different resonances that come from different places in your body. Move the sound up and down between your head and your belly. Have fun with it. Feel all the bones in your head vibrate with the sound. We all resonate to sound on a very deep level. There is a tone exercise in yoga that involves singing, "O, ooo, eee, aaah, ii, aay, oww," and the tones tune up your system. Any vowel will work. If you are tired, this exercise will increase your energy.

If you never sing or hum, ask yourself when you gave it up and why. Who was it who told you not to sing? Do you remember singing as you played alone as a child? I wonder what it is about the natural, joyful sound of children singing that threatens and irritates people so much. A friend of mine has a delightful, joyful child who loves to sing, but her older sister barely lets her get one note out of her mouth before she tells her to be quiet. I think we all have to accept that no matter how perfect our childhood was, there were always people in our lives who wanted to repress and contain our aliveness. The easiest way for them to do that was to restrict our movement and our voices. Let's drown out the voices of our old oppressors and sing or hum our own tune, loud and clear, from the belly.

The Heaven and Earth Breath

This is my favorite. I use it whenever I am out of balance. Read the instructions completely before you start. (There is a lot to learn in this chapter, so take longer than one week if you need to. Practice each breathing exercise and integrate it into your life before you start the next one.)

For this exercise, it is best, especially in the beginning, to stand with your feet firmly planted on the earth. That means real dirt if at all possible, not asphalt or concrete. If this is not possible, vividly remember a time when your two feet were planted on the earth. I recently went to San Francisco for the weekend and, thinking back, my feet didn't touch real earth all the while I was there. Connecting with the earth seems to be a natural consequence of connecting with our bodies. You may find yourself seeking out nature as you become more body-centered.

Close your eyes so that you can internalize your attention. If you are nervous about closing your eyes, drop your gaze down to look at a spot just above the ground. Be comfortable. If you have little trust in your world, acknowledge that and keep your eyes open, gradually working toward shutting out external stimuli.

Breathe into your belly and imagine that with your in-breath you are pulling energy up from the earth through your feet and up your spine to circle in your heart. Send your out-breath deep into the earth, rooting yourself more firmly in this moment. Imagine what earth energy feels like as it travels through you. It will vary with the seasons and the weather. In the springtime, for me, it is a feeling of new growth, of seeds expanding and pushing up through the darkness, seeking the light. In the summer it feels rich, bursting with abundance. In the autumn there is less pushing upward of this energy; fruits are ready for harvest and the energy is beginning to pull back into the earth. Then in winter, it is a slumbering energy, patiently waiting within the soil for new life.

Notice what color the earth energy seems to you—maybe all the greens of growing things springing up from the soil. Perhaps it is the deep rich brown of the earth itself with all the elements that are echoed in our every cell. Or is it the blue of the oceans from which life came? What does earth mean to you? Is it rest and nourishment? Is it support? We are all supported twenty-four hours a day, every second of our life, by the ground beneath our feet, and the force of gravity works to bring us back to the earth in every moment.

We can access the living energy and revitalizing power of the earth by breathing in this way. As you breathe this energy up to your heart, imagine a pink light in your heart growing brighter with each breath.

When you have established a deep connection to the earth, let go of your attention to earth energy, knowing it will keep on flowing by itself. Turn your attention now to the sky above your head. With each new breath, bring the energy of spirit down through the top of your head to your heart. This can be whatever spirit means to you—heaven, angels, Source, Goddess, God, Infinite Wisdom, the Unknown Mystery—it doesn't care what you call it. This energy is usually lighter, clearer, brighter. I imagine it as an unconditionally loving energy.

As it passes your eyes, affirm that you see clearly with the eyes of love. As it passes your throat, affirm that you speak honestly and with love. As it reaches your heart, let it join the earth energy circulating there, and imagine it making the pink light in your heart even brighter. Your heart may actually *feel* different at this point—bigger or with a curious ache. Your heart chakra is opening.

With these
energies
joined
inside you,
you are
limitless.

Now allow yourself to breathe normally and feel yourself completely balanced, as a channel between Heaven and Earth. You may actually feel a current, like a shimmering pulse, passing up and down your spine as you practice this regularly. With these energies joined inside you, you are limitless. Send the pink light from your heart around your body to any part of you that is blocked or in pain. Imagine it flowing like water. Feel it flow all over your body until your cells dance with aliveness. Then if you choose to, you can send this energy out to anyone in your world who needs it. Imagine it flowing from your heart directly to theirs.

Finally, center back into your own heart and take a moment to appreciate yourself for the wonder that you are. Appreciate yourself for the good that you bring into other's lives. Savor and enjoy this step. Don't rush it. When you are ready, open your eyes.

After you get used to the Heaven and Earth Breath, complete the whole process in ten breaths—four from earth, four from heaven, and two for healing. The exercise is like making a friend. It takes more time in the beginning, but after a while, just checking in is enough. For me, the Heaven and Earth Breath is a reality check. When I think the world is not giving me what I want, I check in and get back into balance. You may not remember to do it when you need it most at first, but if you practice it regularly, it will become a wonderful tool for balancing and centering.

If you were uncomfortable with this whole process, just skip it. Some people love it and some don't. Many of my clients were embarrassed at first to do anything that invoked Spirit, but I discovered early in my work that without integrating the force of Spirit with body/mind work, deep change was more difficult. There are so many levels to our awareness, and this breath connects us, in a simple way, to some of the deeper levels operating within our psyche. Meditation is a wonderful tool for those who actually practice it, but I think it is like aerobic exercise—we all know how good it is for us and yet we don't get around to doing it regularly.

With any of the inner work or imagination work in this book, the rule is to "fake it 'til you make it." If you can't possibly imagine earth energy coming up your spine, then just act as if you can. We are all like very exclusive radio receivers. There is an enormous amount of stimuli coming at us at all times and we accept a very narrow range according to our beliefs. We screen out most of it as if it doesn't exist, so allow yourself the freedom to believe that feeling earth energy is possible and you will tune yourself in to the station on which it is playing. We will deal more fully with beliefs and energy in later chapters.

Explorations for the Week

* Learn and practice the three breathing exercises and gradually include them in your repertoire, your toolbox of life. This work on your breath is fundamental to a full and happy life. Love yourself enough to practice until breathing correctly becomes a habit.

* Keep writing in your notebook and keep noticing. The chapters are cumulative. Keep noticing from now on. Keep breathing correctly from now on. The Heaven and Earth Breath, especially, will prepare you for the chapter on energy work.

Resource List

Speads, Carola. *Ways to Better Breathing*. Great Neck, NY: Felix Morrow Publishers, 1986.

Chapter Four

FINDING COMFORT

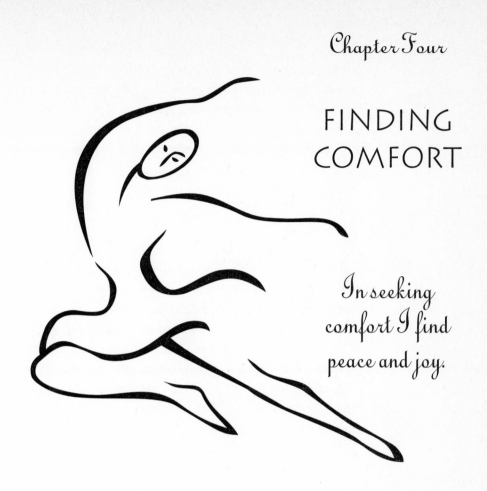

In seeking comfort I find peace and joy.

What image does the word comfort bring to your mind? Lounging in a deep armchair in front of a fire; lying on the beach in the sun; hanging out in your robe and slippers; or maybe being held close in loving arms. We all have different images, but for most of us, there will be some slowing down from our normal pace and, probably, some warmth in our picture.

This chapter will allow you to expand your collection of comfort images. I hope to make the definition of that feeling larger in your experience so that you can feel comfort in your body more often and for longer periods of time. When comfort is clear, a feeling of discomfort, instead of pain, can serve as your body's alarm system.

Can you remember a time when you felt a sense of comfort in doing something you enjoy and do well, without any extra pressure? Pressure of any kind, performance anxiety, drives comfort out and raises our level of stress. Pressure can be external, like time or certain standards that have to be met, or it can be internal, from the high expectations of our inner critic. Wherever the pressure comes from, it erases comfort and pleasure in the task, raises our pulse and our breathing rate, and sets us on edge.

My ideal would be for us to notice those signs of pressure immediately when they occur in our body and develop a response that allows us to adjust back into comfort. It is by this internal monitoring of our comfort level that we can make adjustments in our lives that lead to increased health and well-being. There is an opinion now that a certain level of stress is good for us. I look at it differently. I would say that we need challenge, the excitement of new achievement, and the possibility of success, but we don't benefit from discomfort or stress without that challenge.

Noticing Comfort

The first task is to notice what comfort means to you right now. Throughout the day, make a mental note of when you feel content and totally at ease. Comfort can range from a lack of discomfort to undiluted bliss. Notice that. What about happiness, the goal we are always pursuing? Is happiness the same as comfort for you? What is different about it? Notice the times when your mouth wants to turn up into a smile for no particular reason. Sometimes when I'm driving along my familiar paths I find myself smiling, and a feeling of joy comes over me just because I am alive on this beautiful Earth.

Start to listen for your specific, internal cues for lack of comfort—your breath, your pulse rate, a feeling of edginess in your jaw, tightness in your stomach, a heaviness in your heart, or a need to move away from a situation. Check your eyes for relaxation, and your hands and feet. Check the muscles in your neck, shoulders, and belly. Which cues are the clearest for you? Anxiety is an extreme on the comfort spectrum. What do you do when you are anxious? Do you grind your teeth while you are sleeping? Do you tap your fingers or feet or bite your nails? Do you twist your rings or play with your jewelry? Just notice at this point without trying to change anything.

You are probably very aware, whether you could verbalize it or not, what the body cues are for comfort and discomfort in someone close to you. With one quick glance you can assess the state of mind of your mate, your boss, or your children. Their facial expressions alone probably speak volumes to you. This is a useful skill that women learn through socialization at an early age. I remember, as a child, being fascinated with the changes on the faces of people around me. I could tell exactly how they felt about the people they were with by their minute changes of expression.

Redirect this skill toward yourself. Sneak a look at your own face once in a while, from the inside, without a mirror. You may be surprised at your habitual expression when there is no one else around. Write in your journal a one-word description of what your face conveys. Do you look calm, serene, and happy, or busy, harassed, and troubled?

You may be disturbed to realize how seldom you are truly comfortable and under what a limited range of conditions. Years ago, when someone first pointed out to me that I was actually a nervous wreck passing as a cool superwoman, I was very surprised. It took a few days for me to accept the truth. I was so high-energy all the time and so busy that I really didn't understand what comfort was. I had to stop my normal behavior of tuning out my body reactions to look for it. My attention had been directed completely toward achievement. I was very results-oriented. I could have said immediately what level of well-being my husband or son were experiencing, because their happiness was on my achievement list, but my own was not. I was surprised to find out that I was living on nervous energy.

I had an aunt in England who lived on tea and English biscuits—caffeine and sugar—and I suddenly saw our resemblances. In the same way, a New Yorker friend of mine who visits California always says after a few days, "Oh no! I'm getting mellow. I'd better get back to New York before it's too late." It takes her almost a week to transition into the California lifestyle, but only hours to get sucked back into the energy maelstrom of New York.

It is easier for most people to get hyped up, caught up in stressful circumstances, than it is to unwind. There is a charge of passion and aliveness from dramatic life circumstances that can be addictive. We can become addicted to the adrenaline charge of deadlines and juggling demands. I felt very uneasy at first when exploring comfort because I had to recognize my drama for what it was—an ego defense covering up my discomfort with my life's direction. After a time, you will have a choice about which way you want to go in any moment. Some situations in our lives demand intense energy, but most would really benefit from a deep sense of comfort and peace.

Choosing Comfort

If you find that you are in an anxious, fearful, or upset state, there are specific things you can do to lead yourself back to a greater sense of comfort.

1. If you can lie down, do so. If not, sit in a chair with your back well supported and vertical, both feet on the floor, and your hands separated on your thighs. Breathe deeply into your belly. Move your attention slowly through your body, starting with your toes. Squeeze the muscles in each area as tightly as possible, hold them a moment, and then let go.

Now put your attention on your heart. Breathe in love and breathe out your fear. Set the intention clearly in your mind that you will feel peace in a situation that has bothered you. Notice if you feel comfort with that decision. If not, you may have a desire to continue using the stimulus of the upset for reasons of your own, perhaps to change someone else's behavior. We will deal with that more in the chapter on emotions, but for now see if you can relax into comfort yourself and let the rest of the world be the way it is.

2. Another way to settle into comfort is to relax your face. Our faces hold a lot of tension. They are the windows of our emotional life. Close your eyes and allow your jaw to separate a little. Move your lower jaw in small, slow circles in each direction. Put the middle two fingers of each hand on the joints in front of your ears that move your jaw, the tempero-mandibular joint. Many of us hold chronic tension at this point. You can find it by opening and closing your mouth. Make small gentle circles with your fingers in this location.

    Then, with your index fingers, make small circles at the space between your eyebrows. Gradually move to other places on your forehead until you have gently massaged your entire forehead. In the same slow, gentle way, with small circles, massage all around your mouth. Now, with all your fingers at once, tap very softly all over your face and neck, making the skin glow.

    Lastly, allow your head very gently and slowly to rock back and forth on your neck, looking up to the ceiling and down to your chest. This entire massage can be done in five minutes and it feels so good.

3. This exercise is for your eyes only. In this culture, we are predominately visual learners. So much of our information comes in through our eyes. Prescription glasses and contact lenses are becoming the norm instead of the exception. Push your eyes outward as far as they will go,

as if your life depended on seeing something written on the wall in very small letters. This is the popeye stare. Notice that your eyes do not work independently. Your jaw, your chin, your neck, and your entire back all tighten up as well.

Now allow your eyes to sink back into your head until your head feels soft and loose on your neck. This is the soft gaze. Look around you with the soft gaze and notice that you can see just as clearly, but it seems as if the world outside is coming to you; you are not reaching out to get it.

Go back and forth between the popeye stare and the soft gaze and really become aware of all the differences in the muscles. How far can you trace the tension pattern through your body? When you fully appreciate how tight you feel all over as you reach out with your eyes, you will be able to use your eyes as an indicator for your level of comfort.

We already use this indicator for assessing other people without knowing it. Notice how alarming and upsetting it is to be looked at with the popeye stare and how comforting to be looked at with the soft gaze. As a test, put on your fiercest popeye stare when someone you don't want to talk to approaches you. Use the soft gaze when you want to invite someone's presence. You are a different person when your eyes and face are relaxed.

You are a different person when your eyes and face are relaxed.

I often find that my lack of comfort in the moment has nothing to do with what is happening in my life right now. I am busy in my head, either running tapes of past pain or worrying about my future. As I move through my day, it can be sunny and peaceful and productive, and yet my past and future voices rob me of my sense of comfort. When I wake up to this, I can center myself back into the moment by breathing into my belly, looking about me with a soft gaze, and appreciating the real, live, concrete goodness in my life right now.

It's amazing how much good we can overlook in the present while we preoccupy ourselves with things that may never happen. If the worry thoughts keep returning, I move my body in ways that bring pleasure—dancing, twirling, or just skipping around the room. Try skipping some time when there is no one around. It never fails to make me feel exhilarated, and I laugh like a child.

For one of my clients who was chronically anxious and depressed, the realization that she had some control over her level of comfort was a point of change. She used to say in the jargon that I call therapese, "I don't feel comfortable with that." What she meant was that she didn't like it or she wouldn't accept it. She finally saw and felt that her life had been a refusal to be comfortable unless she won the changes she wanted from others. It wasn't working. When she made the decision to be comfortable, as a gift to herself, her health improved and her resistance to her world melted away. That didn't mean she always liked everything other people chose to do, but she could make her own choices about how to respond without causing herself body discomfort.

Support Versus Challenge

In my work there is always a dynamic balance going on between supporting a client and challenging her. Support has a great deal to do with comfort. I make sure she is comfortable because no one learns well in discomfort; but to learn anything new is a challenge. Feldenkrais work is about learning new options, so I constantly seesaw between accepting a client as she is in this moment, and gently leading her to new choices. In my own life it is the same pattern.

You may remember a time in your life when you felt comfortable and supported by your environment and everything was rolling along smoothly. I call these times of grace the plateaus of life. They are resting places of comfort and support for us to prepare for the challenge ahead. Life doesn't seem to allow us to rest on our plateaus for long. Life happens and, ready or not, we are thrust into the next challenge of our growth.

In small ways that you can observe for yourself, there are opportunities to shift from comfort to challenge. Sitting in front of a television all evening may seem comfortable in one sense, but it saps our impulse toward growth. Our bodies get cranky and sluggish when we sit around for too long. For a deeper, truer sense of body comfort, we have to keep moving.

A client of mine, Sandra, came to me about pains in her legs, hips, and lower back. She had a boring job she hated, sitting at a desk all day. She was short, vertically challenged, as they say, and her feet didn't touch the floor when she sat in her office chair. That is a strange feeling. I tried it on a high stool and I could immediately feel for myself where her pain was coming from. In the evenings, she would lounge on the couch watching television. She felt as if life were passing her by; as if the stream of her life had slowed and she had washed up in an eddy somewhere covered with green algae.

After we had worked together for a while on her pains and she had adjusted her sitting so that she was supported by her feet, she started to feel more powerful. Within a few months, she had moved within her company to a counter job, dealing with people all day, and she was so much happier she could hardly believe it. Without the pains, she was able to walk on the beach for exercise and she took some classes instead of watching television. Her body had been trying to tell her something about her life and she finally heard it.

Comfort in Relation to Others

Notice how the people around you react to your level of comfort with yourself. The real you, the person behind the roles you play, is more accessible when you are comfortable. Most people would rather interact with a person than with a role-player. Relationships warm up, there are fewer misunderstandings and trampled feelings, more smiles, and more sincerity.

Notice also how your level of comfort is regularly affected by the people around you. How many people do you know who convey a sense of personal comfort most of the time? Are these people valuable to you? Are they people you feel safe with? Try to spend more time with people who can model this desirable trait for you.

I have a friend who is always a total joy to be around. I have always wished I were more like Lilli. She is upbeat and energetic and lives much of the time in the now moment. People feel better when she is present. My grandmother was the same way. You can probably remember someone in your childhood who made you feel safe and warm.

Imagine what you would do with your body if you wanted a child to feel safe and comfortable with you. What are the small shifts you would make to appear trustworthy to a child. Among other things, you would probably lower your voice, smile, and become totally present. These are sure clues to a feeling of comfort.

Try an Experiment

In a situation where there are people around you who are anxious or fearful, breathe slowly and deeply into your belly, relax your face, let your eyes rest back into your head, loosen your jaw, and allow a sense of comfort to spread through your muscles. Without saying a word, you are affecting the worried or anxious person for the better. Instead of joining her in her nervous state, you are modeling a more resourceful state. See if you can observe her shift in mood. Having the resource of comfort within is contagious.

Explorations for the Week

❋ Notice when you feel comfortable.

❋ Notice when you do not.

❋ Practice the tools in the "choosing comfort" section—tighten, then relax your muscles; massage your face; exercise your eyes.

❋ Notice your comfort in relation to others.

❋ Pick one person you love and pay attention to how you help them feel comfortable.

❋ Do the same for yourself when you are upset. Be kind and loving to yourself in the same ways.

Resource List

Louden, Jennifer. *The Women's Comfort Book*. New York: Harper Collins Publishers, 1992.

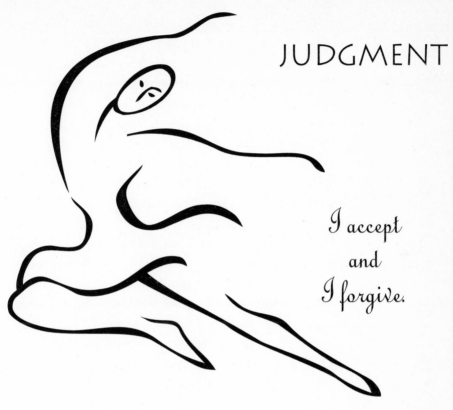

Chapter Five

JUDGMENT

I accept
and
I forgive.

Judging is a deeply ingrained human trait that is absolutely necessary. We need to make hundreds of judgments daily about our options in order to make choices. For instance, if we want to decide whether to wear a raincoat or a sun dress, we make a judgment about the weather and where our day will take us, in order to make a good choice.

There are many times in our day, however, when the simplistic judgments of good and bad, right and wrong, that we learned in childhood, and which are now habitual, operate below the level of our conscious awareness. This kind of judging can often lead to criticism. When negative judgments of self and others become automatic and

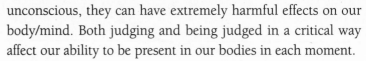

Both judging
and being
judged in a
critical way
affect our
ability to be
present
in our bodies
in each
moment.

unconscious, they can have extremely harmful effects on our body/mind. Both judging and being judged in a critical way affect our ability to be present in our bodies in each moment.

I recently attended a conference on women in mid-life where I overheard two very elegantly dressed women make judgments about everyone who walked in, based on whether their shoes and purses matched. We were a casual, California-style group, and most of us failed the test, including me. In fact half of us were wearing tennis shoes. We spent a large portion of the day discussing all the judgments we and society make about women and the effect of those judgments on our freedom to live our lives. At the end of the day I saw the two women leave and I could see from their body language that they had missed the point.

Whenever we use our appearance, our ethnic group, or our special talents or qualifications to separate ourselves from others, to create a small in-group and a large out-group, we lose. It is only by embracing the enormous spectrum of superficial differences and celebrating them that we can share the underlying unity of who we are as women.

Possibly, the origin of judgment lies within our body structure. On a cellular level, our immune system keeps us healthy by constantly judging. A white blood cell in my body, encountering a particle of any kind, immediately decides whether the particle is a part of my body or an invader; *me* or *not me*. Many of the diseases that have spread in the last thirty years, including cancer, lupus, and AIDS, can be attributed to a breakdown in this immune system; errors in judgment at the level of the cell.

On a societal level, from the family to the species, we also judge constantly; *us* or *them*. When we have decided that a certain group of people is *them*, and therefore not like *us*, we are capable of extreme cruelty toward them, at times to the extent of attempting their annihilation. This is an error in judgment at the level of society. There is always hope that we will become more aware of the larger group—human beings—to which we all belong. Perhaps by acknowledging the deep and biological roots of the human need to judge, we can notice our constant judgments without guilt and with a desire to learn.

Self-Judgment

As women, many of the judgments we have had to deal with our whole lives have to do with our appearance. When you think about it from a heart-centered place, isn't it amazing that ever since we were born the arrangement and shape and size of the features on our bodies have been so incredibly important to our acceptance. Most eyes can see, whether blue or brown, as big as saucers or small. Most noses can breathe and smell, however hooked or bent or wide or lumpy they are. Most mouths can talk and eat no matter how big or small. Yet the mere appearance of these features and their arrangement on our face can make our whole lives happy or wretched.

Aesthetics, the inner appreciation of beauty, isn't even an acceptable excuse because what is considered beautiful in one culture is ugly in another. Do you remember the sixties, when suddenly it wasn't how you *looked* that counted? Odd, nerdy-looking, scraggly, big-nosed, long-haired, fat and thin, young people were accepted for the first time in their lives. Beauty was in the eye of the beholder. Wasn't that an eye-opener? We looked beyond appearances to the beauty within each other. In some cases it took drugs to create that internalized seeing, the seeing with the open heart. Wouldn't it be wonderful if we could forget all of our judgments about ourselves and others, and simply move into acceptance?

This week we will start to become aware of our judgments and how they feel in our body/mind. Since we usually criticize ourselves more harshly and more constantly than anyone else, we will start with self-judgment. We all have an inner critic whose lifework it is to tell us what is wrong with us. This part of our psyche is usually created from our internalized parent, so some of us have tougher, meaner critics than others.

For most of us, the constant voice of the inner critic has been lowered in volume so it often operates beneath our conscious awareness. I have a friend who can't do anything right for her inner critic. If she is working hard on a project, then she is neglecting her children and is a bad mother. If she is playing with her kids, she should be working. This is extreme, but it isn't unusual.

To notice our own daily, regular, familiar judgments about ourselves, it is easier if we bring them to the surface and acknowledge them first. In your notebook, complete the following sentences with as many judgments as you can, without censoring or agonizing over them. Write quickly, and write each one as many times as you need to until nothing else comes up.

✳   My body is too (fat, thin, tall, short, etc.).

✳   My body is not (flexible, attractive, etc.) enough.

✳   What I hate most about my body is (big hips, ugly feet, etc.).

✳   The best age for my body was (sixteen, thirty-five, etc.).

✳   I wish I could, but I can't (swim, ski, write, draw, etc.).

Work fast. Don't dwell on the exercise. We are becoming aware of our judgments so we can STOP making them. Notice the body sensations of self-judgment, but don't get caught up in the feelings that these judgments invoke. These are beliefs and opinions masquerading as fact. We all know people who we consider to be the most beautiful, who are as down on themselves as we are on ourselves. Judgments have little to do with objective reality.

Now for a little balance. Let's write what we like about ourselves. These are judgments too. Again, complete each sentence as many times, and as quickly, as you can.

✳   What I like most about my body is (big eyes, nice hands, etc.).

✳ What others admire about my body is (soft skin, curly hair, etc.).

✳ I appreciate my hands for (sewing, stroking, writing, etc.).

✳ Repeat for legs, eyes, ears, arms, feet, etc.

✳ I am good at (talking, solving problems, painting, etc.).

✳ Other people appreciate me for my talents in (caring, singing, drawing, etc.).

When we are out in the open about our judgments, they can't sneak up on us and undermine us when we are feeling good. Notice from your list how many things you don't like about yourself that will never be different. We can change our hair and even the color of our eyes with the miracles of modern technology, but if we are six feet tall, big-boned, and strong, that's it. That is our body for this lifetime.

We may as well give up our resistance, our kicking and screaming, and accept and appreciate our bodies. Just think about it, our bodies are so good to us. They keep on breathing and fighting germs and carrying us around even under all the extra weight of judgment, shame, and dislike.

On the subject of extra weight, in an informal survey of a large number of women, there were only one or two happy souls who were fully satisfied with their weight. Most women would like to lose at least five pounds. Most of us have the idea that if we could only lose five pounds, it would make a huge difference in our lives. Kind of crazy, isn't it? I now freely confess that I would love to lose ten pounds, but I've decided that I won't wait for that to happen to be happy. I will enjoy myself as I am and then if I lose the weight, great! If not, so what!

Can you remember a time when you really accepted someone? You noticed all their funny little ways and you gave up the craving to change them and just decided to love them anyway. Some of my dearest friends are so different from me. We actually have very little in common. I have moved beyond the space where I want to tell them how to live their lives, and I accept them with all of their interesting choices. *My* life is more interesting just having them in it. If you have never felt that way about a person, maybe you have about an animal. They may bark or shed hair or climb on the couch or get fleas, and you love them anyway. You can do that with your body. It is a wonderful feeling. Not from a place of giving up on yourself, but from true, loving acceptance. Accepting yourself as you are is the only way you can hope to change anyway.

Try an Experiment

 Take a few minutes now and lie down or sit comfortably. Breathe deeply, relax your body, and center your attention at your heart. Remember a time when you held a new baby or a kitten or a flower, and the wonder of life swept over you. Your heart opened and the world felt new and magical and full of unlimited possibilities. Magnify and intensify that feeling, turn up the volume from a one to a ten, until you actually feel your heart responding in some way. Breathe deeply.

In your mind, say the words "I am love" for a minute or so until you can really feel the love, and then send this feeling of love and acceptance throughout your body. Feel the love like a sparkling river flowing into every single cell, and feel your cells start to dance with it. Next send the love directly to a part of your body that you have *not* appreciated in the past. Be open to feeling that part of your body change somehow. Acceptance and love can melt resistance away like the sun on an iceberg. Resistance is the source of most of our pain.

Appreciation of Others

Imagine walking into the biggest library in the world and seeing before you the accumulated wisdom of the ages. Some of the books are huge old leather-bound volumes, fragile and browning at the edges. Some are brightly colored with modern graphics and artwork. Some are almost untouched, clean and stiff, indicating a lack of interest in their contents. Others are very ordinary, unremarkable in any way, except for the wear that speaks of much use. How would you choose your books? Would you judge by appearances alone?

Imagine walking into a garden, well tended, well loved. All about you are flowers of every color, size, and shape; roses in profusion, big bushes and miniatures, sweet-smelling jasmine and lavender, vines and creepers, flowering trees and shrubs. Would you walk down the paths judging the flowers? This one isn't the right shade of yellow; this one is bug-eaten. Or would you just breathe in the wonder of the whole scene, following your nose and eyes from pleasure to pleasure?

Wouldn't it be great to walk into a room full of new *people* with a feeling of trust and acceptance? It is our level of *self*-acceptance that affects our feeling of safety and the number of judgments we make about others. If we are full of fear and insecurity, we will use judgment as a shield and hold it before us as we walk through the room. When you catch yourself doing that, remember the biological origin of this feeling in the reptilian part of your brain. We are bigger than that now, we have evolved.

Put your attention on your heart and move from heart level awareness. Everyone in that room with you has a story to tell. If you approach a person with an open heart and a willingness to listen, you will hear astonishing and moving things. You can drop down beneath the appearances to the real person underneath and share in the joys and sorrows that have formed them.

When you start to notice your judgments of others, it is useful to recognize the small, fleeting changes that occur in your body when you make a judgment. Do you feel safer or smug or self-satisfied or malicious? Does it make you feel bigger or better about yourself to criticize others? Or perhaps, when you catch yourself judging, you instantly feel smaller and guilty, shrinking over in your chest. You probably have experienced both reactions at various times.

One thing you have to remember is that even if you tone down your judgments, you will still have preferences. I don't have any desire to like everything indiscriminately. I will always have my own tastes, likes, and dislikes. There will still be people who I am drawn to and people who do not attract me. I will merely try to stop making other people wrong when they don't share these preferences.

Judging Behaviors

You may find after noticing your judgments for a while that you are judging behaviors as much as appearances. A person may *do* something that bothers you. It is often harder to move into a state of acceptance about actions than appearances. Maybe you could acknowledge that your beliefs and values are different than theirs. Maybe they are behaving in a way that conflicts with their own values and they will eventually feel guilty and stop. Maybe, according to their beliefs and customs, their behavior is perfectly proper and correct. Since you cannot control anyone's behavior but your own, it would be conducive to peace in *your* mind if you could allow others to do the things they do without getting sucked into emotional judgments about them.

Of course, it is different if their behavior is affecting your life directly. Then you will have to negotiate and compromise until a solution is reached. It's amazing, though, how much energy we spend on judging things that are none of our concern, and how often we feel very virtuous about it. We all have such a longing to be right. Being right makes us feel safe and in control of our own lives.

I remember when I first came across the saying, "Would you rather be right or be happy?" It changed the way I looked at disagreements completely. Being right is so isolating. That's why we work so hard to convince others to join us on the side of "right." It's too lonely over there by ourselves.

The problem is that we can be right for ourselves only, not for anyone else. Have you ever listened to someone's problems and seen exactly what they should do to solve them? The solution is always clearer with distance and lack of emotional involvement. How many times have we told our long-suffering friends in struggling relationships to leave their partner, walk away, start fresh? There are more fish in the sea. They don't take our advice most of the time, and that is often a good thing. We all have to move at our own pace and make our own decisions.

Remembering all the times we have been wrong in our own lives could give us a little more humility in making rules of behavior for others. When we judge what is not our business, it sucks our energy away from our own growth. For many people, focusing on what is wrong out there in the world is a good way to avoid the pain of looking at their own lives.

The next time you notice yourself judging someone else's behavior, see if you can generate compassion instead. Take the point of view that they are doing the best they can at this stage in their lives. If they knew how to do it better, they surely would, but it isn't your job to set them straight.

Here is an analogy. Imagine that we are all given a certain amount of money to start with, just like in a Monopoly game. Every thought we have in our lifetime either uses up that money or increases it. Judgments use up money according to their emotional strength: condemnation uses up one hundred dollar bills, mild disapproval uses up one dollar bills. Thoughts of love, acceptance, appreciation, and true compassion increase our money supply according to how intense the emotions are behind the thoughts. How do you think your money supply is lasting? Keep this analogy in mind for one day and see if you are richer or poorer at the end of the day. Given our habit of judgment, it would actually be a miracle if you weren't deeply in debt.

Money is a symbol for energy, so it is not hard to imagine that an appreciative thought might build up our energy and a judgmental thought might deplete us. For me, this is very clear when I feel my body reactions. When I make a lot of negative judgments, my body feels draggy and listless. When I am open and accepting and loving, my body feels great.

Feeling Judgments

How do *you* react in your body when you are being judged? Do you shrink a little or pull your shoulders forward to hide your heart? Or does your chin come up and your back arch? Do you immediately react with resentment when people criticize you? How does resentment feel in your body? For me, resentment ties up my tongue and my face. I can't speak freely or smile until I have dealt with it. It's not a productive feeling.

We see the non-productivity of this behavior most clearly when we judge a child and see her reaction. Actually, any form of judgment usually brings our own inner child into play instantly. When your boss criticizes you, do you feel four years old again? If you were a "good" four-year-old, you may feel your chin trembling and a desire to cry. If you were a rebellious four-year-old, you may feel your fists clenching and yearn to kick or hit. From this viewpoint, you have no skills or tools that can serve you. It is necessary to shift back into the consciousness of the adult to evaluate the criticism honestly.

Often, those of us who were most harshly judged as children, judge others most severely as adults. I have a friend who was constantly wanting as a child. She never measured up to her mother's expectations. She made up her mind never to talk to her own children in any critical, put-down way, but to encourage them in everything they did. She does well with that most of the time, but on a bad day, when she is rushed and stressed, she sometimes catches her mother speaking through her, saying the exact words she swore she would never say. She can stop herself very quickly when she sees the clear effect of her words on her children's body posture and their faces, and she can remember how she felt in her own younger body.

Changing Judgments

After you have noticed your judgments for a time, they will diminish in frequency and intensity, merely as the gift of awareness. If you would like to shift more actively into a positive way of viewing your world, here are some tools.

First comes acceptance, as usual. We don't have to be ashamed of how judgmental we are. It is a skill we learned from society, and most of us learned it very well. We are not intrinsically negative or worthless because we learned it well. Now we are at the fulcrum of change. To succeed in the next century, society needs different skills. First we learn and integrate, then we teach others.

One Feldenkrais tool I find very useful is exaggeration. Every time you find yourself judging yourself or others, go for it. Step it up. Exaggerate outrageously. You aren't just having a bad hair day, you could scare off a vampire. When you do it to the extreme, you get absurd and funny. Most of us obsess over faults that are so minor no one else ever notices them, so we are already exaggerating and just aren't aware of it.

The next tool is appreciation. Every time you look in the mirror and say something nasty to yourself, consciously change channels and find something to praise yourself for. Anything will do. Your eyes may be clear and sparkling; your creative work may be flourishing; your house may be clean. Think of small things and make them clearly positive. No buts. Not, my teeth are white, *but* I have a lot of fillings. Be kind to yourself. Give yourself the loving appreciation you would give a small child or your wonderful old grandmother. Better yet, give yourself the appreciation you always wished someone else would give you.

Every time you feel your worth has not been acknowledged, do it for yourself. Praise yourself for every completed task, every improvement in your life, every effort you make to become more of the wonder that you are. Praise yourself just for being you. There is magic in this.

Teach yourself to appreciate others in the same way. Every time you judge an appearance, find something about the person to praise. This is not insincerity. It is just looking through a different set of lenses. We are all so creative. We can always find *something* to praise. If you are judging someone's behavior, find something else they do that you can commend. No one does it *all* wrong. We are such a mixture. Even our worst enemy has good qualities. Now it is your job to find them.

Go into your heart and look with eyes of compassion on people and situations you are tempted to judge. If this is more difficult with certain people in your life, then actually imagine yourself face to face with your adversary. In your mind's eye, walk over and stand beside her, see with her eyes and feel what she is feeling. You could then ask yourself whether you might have the ability to act in the same way given the right set of circumstances.

All possibilities exist within us. I have some beliefs written out and taped on my bathroom mirror. One is: *People are either speaking from love or calling for help.* By joining people on their side for a moment and being willing to share their fear and pain, we can answer their cry for help. Try it. You will feel an overall difference in the quality of your life.

Explorations for the Week

✳ Notice your judgments about yourself first, and change them to appreciation.

✳ Practice the love exercise on page 58 every day.

✳ Notice your judgments about others, and allow yourself to

feel compassion for them. From a compassionate, loving space, you may be able to say something that would really help them.

* Notice how you feel when you have been judged by someone in your life. What do you think would have worked better to help you.

* In your notebook, explore how a world without judgment would look.

* Explore the saying, "People are either speaking from love or calling for help."

* Be especially kind to yourself this week.

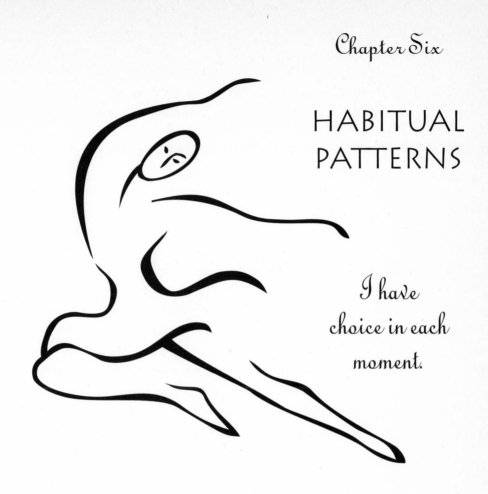

Chapter Six

HABITUAL PATTERNS

*I have
choice in each
moment.*

Habitual patterns are those things we do without thought, except to wonder at times why everybody else doesn't do the same thing. These patterns usually have both a physical and a psychological or emotional component. There are habitual patterns that are cultural, such as being friendly toward strangers; there are habitual patterns that are gender differentiated, such as women being ready to give comfort when someone looks upset; and there are idiosyncratic patterns you may have that you think are the norm, such as finishing other people's sentences, but that drive your friends wild.

This week, we are going on the hunt for these habitual patterns in ourselves and others. Once again, the object of the game is to have choice. If our habits are running us without our awareness, we don't have choice.

One of the major premises in this book is that the more we learn about ourselves and the more options that are available to us, the richer our lives will be. If we see the brain as an incredibly complex network of connections, anything new we learn creates a new neural pathway. Instead of traveling on the old, rutted paths of our habitual patterns, we will be striking out and making new tracks within our brain, which will be available to us forever.

Usually, we notice patterns in our daily lives only when someone remarks on them. Otherwise, we go merrily on our way, thinking we are the same as everyone else. When a person comments on our habitual optimism, or our way of interrupting all the time, or our habit of looking for the best in people, we become aware that we are different. We look at the world in our own special way.

An easy way to discover some of your habitual patterns for yourself is to notice whenever you say, "I always" or "I never." Both of these statements are limitations, and that is what most habits are. It saves us time to have habits. If we had to be fresh and new in every moment, we would never get anything done; but habit also limits our experience.

For example, my mother has been going to a group meeting for years. Everyone sits in the same place each time they meet. It is easier because they don't have to decide each time where they want to sit and they don't have to risk hurting anyone's feelings, but my mother is limiting her experience of the group. She knows that it would cause quite a stir if she were to cross the large room and sit with the women on the other side. She is conscious of this habitual pattern, but many of the women in the group are not. Sometimes she moves up one or two seats and watches the consternation of the person she has displaced. Have you ever done that?

Being territorial is a very common human pattern. We stake out our claim to a certain chair or spot and get upset when others don't realize it is ours. That reminds me of the women in Las Vegas who play the slot machines. They lay claim to a whole row of slots and you could suffer grievous bodily harm if you put a nickel in one of *their* machines by mistake.

Another way to bring your own patterns to awareness is to notice when you are surprised or shocked by someone else's behavior. Obviously, their pattern is different than yours, and your own is so familiar to you that you think it is universal. You also probably think it is *right*.

In England, where I grew up, there was consensus about many of our daily behaviors. We all learned early the *proper* way to do everything and the social perils of deviation. In the wonderful melting pot of ethnic groups here in the United States, there is less conformity to tradition and more freedom to discover new patterns for ourselves. Trying something new could even be said to be an honored American pattern.

Physical Patterns

We have many purely physical habits that are so ingrained we are unaware of them: the way we walk and talk and laugh, for example. Usually, any member of a family can tell which other family member is approaching from the sound of their footsteps alone. Science has discovered that it is not only our fingerprint that can identify us beyond doubt, our voiceprint is also unique. Even within a family, our voices are all usually very dissimilar. The way we hold our jaw to speak is the result of our own particular view of the world. Some habits can be changed as soon as they are brought into awareness and others cannot. We can change our accent with a little work, but our unique voiceprint will still give us away.

One physical pattern I changed recently was squinting in the sun. I was getting a crease, like a frown, between my eyebrows and starting to look like a grouch, so I quickly learned not to squint. As we get older, the lines on our faces tell a story about our lives, through our habitual patterns of expression.

Gravity is a mixed blessing as we age. As our mouths start to droop toward our feet, it takes a very optimistic outlook on life to look habitually cheerful, if, indeed, we would even want to. What does *your* habitual expression say about you?

One of the most prominent physical habit patterns is our choice of right or left hand dominance. Moshe Feldenkrais thought that if we would become ambidextrous, we would be adding an enormous new capacity to the brain.

Try doing some less important tasks with your non-habitual hand this week, maybe brushing your hair or teeth. It may feel awkward at first, but it could help to equalize the wear on your wrist and shoulder joints as well as create new pathways in your brain.

Have you noticed that most people hold one shoulder higher than the other? Figure out for yourself which shoulder is higher on most people, the shoulder of their dominant hand or the other one.

We also have a dominant standing leg. We stand with most of our weight on one leg most of the time, and we usually move out first with the other leg. We choose to jump or climb steps with the moving leg first. See if you can alternate legs and stand with your weight on your moving leg more. You will gradually come to feel more balanced.

As people become upset or anxious, the first physical habitual pattern to kick in will be breathing into their upper chest. If the anxiety continues, you will notice all kinds of unconscious worry movements—biting their nails, compulsive eating, scratching, shaking, twitching, tapping hands or feet, etc. When people are happy and content, these behaviors are absent.

Early Bird or Late-Comer

Are you habitually late or early for every appointment? Do you often go out with someone who is the opposite? This is a surprisingly frequent cause of disagreements.

Notice which is your habitual preference without making it good or bad. Experiment with changing. If you are always early, pick an occasion when you won't drastically affect anyone else, and try to arrive late. You may find this very difficult at first. Persist until you manage it, even if you experience some anxiety.

This is an old childhood pattern, and the reason for the anxiety usually has little to do with the present. The young age at which this pattern was learned is the reason it polarizes people so much. Our parents and teachers always wanted us to be on time and we were punished in various ways for being late. Some of us are complying tenaciously and some of us are still rebelling thirty years later.

If you are a habitual late-comer, give yourself permission to stop the rebellion and try being early. Once again, you may find it astonishingly difficult. People I know trick themselves with fast clocks or leave with time to burn, and still somehow manage to arrive late. Notice your feelings about it. Are you irritated that people get so hung up about time? Is it depressing to always be upsetting people with your lateness? Go back and forth between being early and late and see what feels comfortable for you. Bring the whole pattern into conscious awareness. Remember your parents' attitudes toward time. Which parent are you most like?

I am an early bird partly because I am usually eager to get on with life. If it's good, let me at it. If it's bad, let's get it over with. After experimenting for a while, I felt that I had a choice. When I am late now, I don't get anxious about it. I sometimes even choose to be late for certain events, especially in California. When I arrived on time, I often found my hostess in the shower or I was enlisted to help cook dinner.

Another side benefit of this experiment is that I no longer get angry when other people are late. I used to think they were inconsiderate and rude, and I took it very personally when they were late. Now I just do what I need to do—leave without them or wait without rancor.

Helping

There are many gender-specific patterns that have a psychological component as well as a physical one. A very common pattern with women concerns helping. *We are just such helpful people!* When I have a male client for Feldenkrais work and I pick up an arm or a leg, they generally lie there like the dead and let me get on with it. Not so with women. As soon as I reach out to pick up their arm, there it is in my hand. As soon as they think they know where I am going to go with it, there it is.

In Feldenkrais, it is important to *not* help, to be a passive learner, but it is no use saying that at first. Women have a hard time *not* helping. It's a new skill and they have to learn it. This deeply ingrained pattern is important to examine because some of us get so little true rest. Even if no one needs anything at the moment, we are on the alert on a subconscious level for when they do.

It is very common among English women I know, that as soon as a desire escapes the lips of her husband or children, she is on her way to gratifying it. If their loved ones don't speak up, they will constantly ask, "Does anyone want a cup of tea? Is anyone hungry? Don't you need a sweater?" Maybe it is more common in England, but I have seen it often enough here in the United States also.

A good time to notice this pattern is at mealtimes. If you are sitting at the table and a member of your family wants something, do you jump up and get it? Are you always asking your family if there is anything they want or need? Are you genuinely happy to be of service in these small ways, or are you often resentful?

It is often not a positive thing to do tasks for others that they could do for themselves. The help comes from a loving heart, but it does not encourage self-reliance. A friend of mine never taught her children to help out with the household chores when they were small. Now they are teenagers and she can't wait for them to grow up and leave. They take her work of making their home comfortable completely for granted.

The point is that your body will wear out sooner if you are constantly ready to act on other's whims. In answering our own desires, our bodies can fully relax between the movements we make to satisfy these desires. That is the way our bodies were designed, to move and to rest fully between movements. When we are at the beck and call of others, this complete relaxation no longer occurs.

Sometimes a readiness to act is much more tiring than completing the action would be. Have you ever been in a hospital waiting room while someone you love is ill? You want to help so badly but there is nothing you can do. It is exhausting. You are probably more tired than the nurses who are doing the actual work.

When I asked one client, who was very stiff, to watch for the helping habit in her life, she replied that she had no children and a loving husband, and she did not have that pattern. During the next week, she was surprised to discover that she certainly did. It would be unusual for a woman not to have it after the socialization of so many centuries. Look for this pattern in your own life this week.

In answering our own desires, our bodies can fully relax between the movements we make to satisfy these desires.

Feminine Patterns

In addition to the helping pattern, we have many other habitual patterns that are gender differentiated. Of course, we are all a blend of feminine and masculine energies, and many women have a lot of male patterns in their repertoire. In fact, we have been encouraged since the women's liberation movement to acquire common male patterns in order to make it in the business world. Being competitive, being linear, and following rules are patterns common to men that women have had to learn.

When men and women are complaining about each other, we can notice some opposite patterns. Women will say men are inflexible, while men will say women are too changeable. Women say men are non-verbal, while men say women talk too much. Once again, the peaceful solution is to recognize and celebrate our differences. Who would want to live in a world full of clones?

Think of a feminine pattern you have, and try not to get caught up in it this week. For example, are you a comforter? Do you need everyone in your world to be happy and content all the time? Do you mediate all the quarrels and comfort the wounded? Are you a woman people can count on to make *their* troubles your own? Do you ignore your own need for comforting?

Try putting yourself first for a week. Allow people their unhappiness. No one can be happy all the time. This is a world of duality. Too much of the same emotion is boring. Accepting someone's negative feelings without trying to help them or change them is a real gift. What you learn about yourself will be interesting. Change job patterns the same way if you haven't already. You mow the lawn and take out the garbage, and teach your partner to do your chores.

Nurturing, cleaning, caring, sympathizing, cooking, picking up after, helping, finding, comforting, joining, sharing, being efficient, mediating, remembering, being spontaneous, intuitive, and sensitive are some feminine patterns. Many of them are actually the skills of a homemaker, and a lot of younger women have fewer of these patterns. An old lady friend of mine says of young women today, "They don't cook, they don't clean, they don't do laundry, and they have sex without a ring. Why in the world would anyone want to marry them?" Luckily for the continuation of society, there is the old habitual pattern of bonding and partnering deep in our genetic programming, and it has nothing to do with how well you wash shirts.

Exploring New Patterns

We all have hundreds of habitual patterns we can pay attention to. It is funny how just recognizing them often makes us feel better. I used to feel very upset when my partner and I had a silly fight after a period of closeness. I finally realized that it was a habitual pattern of his to create distance in that way when we got too close. When we brought it out in the open, we no longer needed to fight. He would just say that his bliss tolerance level had been exceeded and he needed some space.

If a close friend has a pattern you don't have, try it out. Pick a positive pattern at first, something like jumping out of bed wide awake and happy. It's odd how we don't think we have choice about something like that. Then try the opposite, pushing the snooze button ten times, snuggling back under the covers, refusing to think about the day ahead, and finally getting up at the last minute. See which pattern works better for you.

I had a sleep pattern for years that required absolute quiet and darkness before I could sleep. It was a real bother. I didn't realize back then that I could change it. I thought that was just the way I was. Fortunately, I was smart enough to teach my son, Tim, to sleep anytime, anywhere. I finally outgrew my pattern on a year-long trip to South America under somewhat grueling conditions. On that trip, if I hadn't given up the need for quiet and darkness, I would never have had a good night's sleep. By the end of the trip I could sleep on buses, trains, restaurant seats, hard beds, even next door to a riotous celebration.

Now I have the same pattern as Tim; when I am tired, I sleep wherever I am. Life is so much simpler. What we have to remember is that we all have a list of preferences a mile long and we often create habitual patterns around them. Just remember that you created your preferences and your habits, and you can change them if they no longer suit you.

If you are ready for a challenge, pick a habitual pattern a friend has that has always bothered you. Explore the pattern for yourself. Not with a feeling of vengeance—I'll show her how it feels—but with a desire to learn. The pattern obviously works for her on some level; maybe you can learn from it.

Unreliability has always been one of my biggest aggravations. What I learned from my exploration was the sweet sense of freedom I could feel when I forgot everyone else's plans and needs. It was such a carefree feeling at first. I knew that my friend didn't do it on purpose to irritate me. She is just better at forgetting than I am. I finally came to realize that I had been painfully super-conscientious. Of course, I always subconsciously expected a payoff for my goodness and got very resentful when no one noticed.

I learned a lot from exploring many facets of unreliability, but after a while, I decided that the pattern didn't feel natural for me. I didn't feel as connected as before. The good part is that I no longer get irritated with my friend for having that pattern. I am now more willing to double check our arrangements with her in case she forgets. Another funny thing is that I seemed to be surrounded by people who were unreliable and forgetful before, and now, if I am, I don't notice it.

Acting Out Opposites

You have probably noticed by now that many of our habitual patterns occur in pairs—early bird/late-comer, reliable/unreliable, etc. In relationships, and within families, it is not coincidental that most conflict occurs around these polarities.

It is almost as if we decide which roles we will play when we first meet. "Okay, I'll take dependent, but you have to take authoritarian, and you can take moody too. I'll be merrily empty-headed and you can be serious."

Sometimes this division of roles can last a long time, but eventually, one of the partners changes and upsets the balance. Then the unspoken negotiation has to start all over again.

Examine your life with brutal honesty and see if you can decide which side of some of these polarities you are on:

Giver/receiver

Shy/outgoing

Quiet/gregarious

Meticulous/careless

Obedient/rebellious

Tactful/outspoken

Child/parent

Rational/intuitive

Affectionate/cold

Honest/dishonest

Loose/tight

Optimistic/pessimistic

Winner/loser

Pleaser/rebel

Clever/stupid

With different people in our lives, we often act out different sides of the polarity. We will probably act in a different way around men than among women. If you act like a winner with some people and like a loser with others, ask yourself what it is about the relationship that evokes that behavior from you.

Notice if you have a strong reaction to one of the polarities, dishonesty for example. Most of us would like to think that we are honest women, but I'm certain there is some small corner of your life in which you are less than totally truthful. The value of this experiment is to discover for ourselves that we can be anything we choose, if only for five minutes.

Pick one polarity that you are used to playing and act out its opposite. Other people will have to adjust their behavior and they may resist and try to force you back into the old pattern. To experience the new pattern successfully, you have to feel in your belly how it would feel and then allow your body to act it out. A loser has different body posture than a winner. If you forget how the role feels, go back to your belly and imagine being in the role until it starts to come naturally.

This may not be easy. You may think you can't possibly be gregarious; you are shy and that's all there is to it. Not true. You have been around gregarious people and have seen this trait modeled, so somewhere in your body/mind that pattern is ready to be expressed. Your body/mind knows more than you can possibly imagine. You are truly unlimited in the roles you can play, so go ahead and audition for some new choices. Have fun with this exercise.

Beliefs

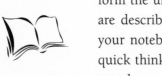

Habitual patterns are usually based on beliefs we hold about reality. We aren't always conscious of our beliefs, but they form the underpinnings of our behaviors. Imagine that you are describing yourself to someone. Write a description in your notebook. Start with, "I am …" For example: I am a quick thinker, a morning person, somewhat reserved, often moody, etc.

Everything you wrote is a belief you hold about yourself. Have you ever had a belief about yourself that changed drastically? If you did the work in the previous section, maybe you have already changed some beliefs. I used to say I had no musical aptitude. I wished I did, but I didn't, just like I don't have green eyes. Of course, there was a reason I believed that. A frustrated teacher had told me so when I was eight or nine. A friend pointed out to me some time ago that I loved music, I could tell a good note from a bad one, a tenor from a bass, and I had as much musical aptitude as the average. Since then I have even sung in a choir.

Any belief can be changed. We change an enormous number of beliefs about ourselves as we grow up. Think of some beliefs you had about yourself as a teenager that you just grew out of. I believed for years as a pre-teen and young teenager that I would never get a date. Here I am two husbands later.

Most beliefs, like the habitual patterns they create, limit us in some way. I decided long ago to choose some primary beliefs for myself that give me more freedom.

I believe I am limited only by my interests. That means I'll never be like Georgia O'Keefe or Beethoven because I am not willing to put all my time and energy into art or music; but whatever interests me I can learn and do well.

My life is a guided journey. The habitual pattern that comes out of this belief would be learning from everything that happens to me whether it feels good or bad at the time.

Think of beliefs, and the habitual patterns that come from them, as the roles you have chosen for yourself, or that maybe your parents chose for you. In the hypothetical example of being somewhat reserved, the habitual pattern of behavior would be to hang back, not join in, not smile much, not be open and forthcoming, not trust people readily, and to be cautious. Do you see how limiting that is? If all our life is but a stage, as Shakespeare said, maybe we would want to play that role for a while to see how it feels, but surely not forever.

Go back to the description you wrote about yourself and look at the roles you are choosing to play. If some of the roles are too limiting for you, pick some new beliefs, try out some different habitual patterns, and write your own script. *This is your life*.

Explorations for the Week

* Notice your habitual patterns and experiment with the opposite.

* Pick a pattern a friend has that you like, and try it out.

* Pick a pattern that irritates or bothers you, and try it out.

* Notice masculine and feminine patterns around you.

* Try acting out at least one of the polarities listed.

* In your notebook, do the work in the beliefs section.

* Write some new, non-limiting beliefs for yourself and post them where you can see them.

* Read what you have written so far in your notebook and give yourself credit for the changes in awareness you have accomplished.

We are about halfway through the workbook at this point. Are you still practicing the breathing exercises? Are you more aware of your bodily comfort in an ongoing way? Is this book working for you? Is there a way you can make it work even better?

Uncover your beliefs about change, growth, and learning. If you have a limiting belief that learning is difficult, for example, consider changing it. One of mine is: Learning and growing make life exciting and worthwhile.

Resource List

Tanenbaum, Joe. *Male and Female Realities*. Costa Mesa, CA: Robert Erdman Publishers, 1990.

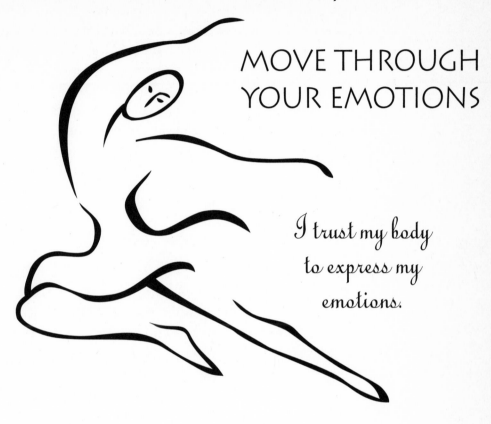

Chapter Seven

MOVE THROUGH YOUR EMOTIONS

*I trust my body
to express my
emotions.*

oes it feel to you sometimes as if your emotions are like wild dogs that have you by the throat and won't let go; or like germs floating around in your environment looking for a host to feed on? I have some good news and some bad news. The good news is that *we* are the creators of all of our emotions. The bad news is that we can't *blame* our emotions on anyone else. They are created out of the raw material of our lives and it is only in our resistance to having them move through us that we experience pain.

Emotions are energy in motion. They are designed to wash through our body/mind like the waves on the seashore, leaving us clean and new. We can't pick

It is
impossible
to feel bliss
if we are
unwilling
to experience
despair.

and choose which emotions we are willing to express. When we try to shut out negative feelings, or block their flow through our bodies, all our emotions are affected. The blocks gradually accumulate in our body/mind over the years, leading to stiffness and pain. It is impossible to feel bliss if we are unwilling to experience despair. I read recently that testing the immune systems of people before and after experiencing strong emotions revealed that the immune system was strengthened by *both* positive and negative emotions. It is better for us to feel grief than to not feel at all.

The Witness State

Since the second chapter, we have been learning to notice thoughts or habits that we have, or movements that we make. We have been learning to create the witness state. The witness is the part of us that is separate from our behaviors and can merely witness the behavior. You can clearly distinguish by now the witness from the inner critic who watches in order to judge you. The witness is the part that can watch you living your life and be interested and curious about you in a loving, yet impartial way. You are much more than your behaviors and emotions, and the witness recognizes that.

The witness belongs to the larger "I," or the Higher Self, who sees *all* of the imaginable possibilities of your life and watches you choose the paths you want to explore. The Higher Self loves you unconditionally and sees clearly how every lesson in every moment of your life leads you on toward home—the alignment of body, mind, and Spirit. The truth is that we are not the movie that is playing out right now in our lives. We are the screen on which the movie plays. We could choose to play another movie any time or we could make a decision that would change our movie forever.

Have you ever dreamed of running away from your life and starting fresh? As a child I longed to run away and join the circus and become a trapeze artist. At other times in my life, I have considered signing up on a sailboat crew going around the world or joining Mother Theresa. Whenever I consider these possible escapes from the movie that I am creating right now, that has become somehow unsatisfying or boring, I feel better about my life. I can more willingly make the small changes I need to make to move on.

So many of us sometimes feel trapped in our lives, but the truth is that we all have choice. There is always a way to run a new movie on your screen if you only want to badly enough. We tend to identify so completely with our roles that we forget sometimes that that is what they are, just roles. It seems to be an ironic twist of fate that natural disasters and wars seem to shake us out of our limited roles and teach us about our resources and capabilities in a way that often surprises us. Crisis often evokes our better selves. We forget our small, daily concerns and rise to the occasion. Within families, long-standing differences and grudges are often given up in the face of severe illness or death.

So what does all this have to do with emotions? I have found that women often have a resistance to believing they can change their emotions at will anytime they want to. Women identify with their emotions in a way that forgets the existence of the witness. You may be playing out sadness or depression in your movie right now, but your witness can easily remember a time of peace or joy or excitement or elation.

We have the whole gamut of emotions at our disposal. Our repertoire of emotions as human beings is vast. There is not an emotion that has ever been felt by a human that we don't have access to, and the miraculous thing is, they are all transitory. We can't hang on to any of them without making ourselves sick. Emotions are designed to move through us like clouds on a summer sky and enrich our lives as they pass.

Emotions
are designed
to move
through us
like clouds
on a summer
sky…

Moving with Feelings

The trick to having your emotions flow through you in a way that energizes your life is to move your body with the feeling. In order to prevent feeling pain, we generally tighten our muscles and restrict our movement. The first thing we do in an uncomfortable situation is hold our breath, and then we tighten our shoulders and our bellies. The fight or flight mechanism is well-known, but the third alternative, to freeze, is actually more common to women than is acknowledged.

Whenever I have been hurt deeply, I freeze into a slightly curled over position, protecting my heart, and I go blank. I couldn't think of a creative solution to my difficulty in this position if you offered me a million dollars. Fortunately I have learned to force myself to move, to get up and walk around, and breathe, so I can come back to life. Coming back to life means that I will have to feel the pain, cry or yell it out of my body, but I have learned that it is worth it to me. My body no longer carries the disappointments and misunderstandings of my life.

The next time you are conscious of deep feeling while alone, notice where in your body this feeling resides. Now breathe into that place and move in whatever way your body wants to. Your body is infinitely wise. It knows what movements will heal you. Freezing, denial, and repression can never heal you. If they could, heaven knows, we would all be healthy. There isn't a woman alive who hasn't tried them all, over and over again. You may be afraid to try this new behavior. *Do it anyway.* A voice may tell you that you are stupid or that you can't feel anything in your body. Go inside and watch. Find the part of you that you are holding tight against the flow of emotion. Some part of your body is waiting to move, to squirm, to wriggle, to run away, to scream, or to hit.

We have been taught to repress the healthy expression of our feelings since we were small children. Watch a healthy, small child express disappointment sometime. Her face clouds over, her chin trembles, she starts to cry. If the disappointment is severe enough and she isn't interfered with in some way, she may throw herself on the ground and sob. After a short while, the energy of the emotions will wane and she will get up and get on with her life. Only when children are interfered with, bribed in some way not to feel their feelings, not to move through their pain, will the emotion persist in their body memories or haunt their dreams.

Pain, sadness, and anger that is repressed and not permitted to move through you, will turn into depression. Some of us have had depression of such long standing, like an ever-present blue note running through our lives, that we have completely forgotten what the original pain was about. Psychotherapy works to retrieve the buried memories and we sometimes reach a broad intellectual understanding of the roots of our problems, yet it often doesn't help.

Until we have moved the pain out of our body memory, we don't move on in our lives. I really believe that it is unnecessary to recover the memory of every negative thing that ever happened to us. If your inner wisdom decides you need to remember specific events in order to heal, it will bring them up while you are moving.

If you are moving through your feelings organically, you remember only what you have the inner strength to integrate and deal with. Don't get caught up in the drama of finding out exactly *who* did *what* to you *when*. It doesn't help you get on with being in the NOW moment in a joyful way. You can get caught up in the innocent victim role all over again. Most of us have been playing out that role for years already. Let's set the intention to give that one up. When we stop blaming our past, we have to take responsibility for our lives as they are right now, and if we don't like our lives, *we can change. We* are the center of the point of power.

Until we have
moved the pain
out of our
body memory,
we don't
move on in
our lives.

Exaggerate

The next time you feel a deep emotion that seems to be recurrent, like always being disappointed when someone doesn't call, even though you know they are forgetful or busy, find yourself a safe place to do some work. Rerun the incident in your mind and notice where you are feeling some sensation in your body. Exaggerate whatever sensations you are feeling and put words to them.

If your throat is tightening, tighten it more, grab it with your hands and say what you are doing to yourself. "I will not let you speak." You are doing it anyway, you may as well verbalize it. If your hands tighten into fists, do it more. For me this one says, "I hate you!" If your feet itch to kick out, do it more. If you fold over into a fetal position, do it more. My words for this one are, "I wish I'd never been born." Very dramatic. That is what we are looking for here—drama—even melodrama. Overact. Be shameless. We are all actors after all. Just keep moving or speaking what you are doing.

If you are numbing out or getting stuck, go back to the provoking incident and re-run it in your imagination. If you are feeling stupid or embarrassed, acknowledge that feeling and keep on acting out anyway. Notice if you remember a time long ago when you felt just the same way. If nothing comes to you, that's fine too. Your intention is to experience the drama so completely that when you are done, it is over with forever.

If you think you are done and then you say something in your head a while later that gets you going again, start over. Notice what you said to bring it back. My words usually are, "It will never be the same." Whenever I am grieving a loss of any kind, I make sure to say those words over and over, and start crying and sobbing all over again, until finally I say it and my whole body responds with, "That's okay. So what. You'll be fine." Then I know I am really done. Of course, if you are grieving the loss of someone dear to you, it may be necessary to repeat this process many times, but each time you will come to a clearer space in your letting go.

When I am dramatizing grief, I will eventually come to a place of peace. When I am exaggerating anger, I usually come to a place of laughter. I hit the pillows or imagine cutting my adversary up into small pieces. If the person is an authority figure, I imagine them in ridiculous situations. I get very creative with my vengeance until finally I laugh until my ribs hurt. Don't feel guilty about wishing your adversary harm. We are not so powerful that we can hurt people with our thoughts in such a short space of time. Harboring long-standing resentment hurts the people in our lives much more.

This process of clean anger usually leads me to deep forgiveness of my adversary's actions, and my own, and I can see us both more clearly and gain insight that will head off future misunderstandings. Most people out there in the world who make us angry are just triggering our childhood pain anyway. That is why I rarely confront anyone when I am upset. I own my feelings and work on them by myself first; then I am clearer about what needs to be said to resolve the situation without blame.

Blaming someone else may be ego gratifying in the short term, but it never works to make me feel better in the long run. When I have resolved an upset in this organic way, I feel bigger, my heart feels open and warm, I feel good all over. When I am still in the grip of blame and justification and control, I can often win because I am clever with words, but my heart is still small and it still hurts. Don't you know that feeling? To me it says I'm not done yet, there is still more work to do.

If you go through the whole process and come to a clear space and the person you are upset with is still back at the level of the upset, that's okay. We can do our work, but we can't do theirs for them. Give them some space and love and they will either come around or they won't. It isn't important any more. The child in us often fears that our anger or sorrow is bottomless and endless, but when we do this moving process we always come to the bottom if we act out enough.

*… we have
the ability
to heal
our past
while we deal
creatively
with
our present.*

We may fear that our anger will lead us to kill someone, but anger stored up in our body cells will more likely end up killing us. By working alone on our anger, we can take responsibility without hurting anyone else. In the clearing out of every deep emotion in this way, as we feel it, we have the ability to heal our past while we deal creatively with our present.

Timing your Emotions

It seems as if it is rare in our busy lives to be free to deal with our emotions as they come up. Something may trigger old pain or an over-reaction in the middle of our workday or in a place where we are expected to act professionally. To be true to our feelings in the moment is a wonderful way to live, but it is idealistic. In the real world, we often have to put our emotions on hold until a more appropriate time. I believe that as long as you promise yourself to deal with the emotion later, and keep your promise, you will not lock the blocked emotion in your body tissue.

For example, if you become upset at something that happens during a business meeting, you have three choices. You can protect yourself so completely that you don't even hear it. I did that for years. When I was home alone I often realized that I was sad and forlorn, and I would have to re-run my day to discover the reason.

The second choice is confrontation. You can hash out the disagreement right there and then. Most of us have so much old baggage of hurts and upsets that can be triggered innocently by the behavior of a colleague that this is a risky choice. When you are upset, you are revealing much more about yourself than you realize.

The third choice is to hear the words, witness and acknowledge your reaction, and immediately promise yourself to work on it later alone, and then get back to the business at hand. Upset of any kind will trigger our child personas within, and the last thing most women want to do is to relate to colleagues and bosses with all the tender feelings of a four-year-old.

If you think you cannot put your feelings on hold in this way, try to remember a time when you were forced to do so. In emergency situations, I have often been the person who handles the crisis perfectly, only to collapse later. We do have choice. Have you ever been sad over a loss, maybe a death, when the whole world looks gray to you, and someone takes you to a funny movie? You find yourself laughing and forgetting your pain. When you walk out of the theater it settles back on your shoulders.

When my father died, I had to continue working although I wanted to just curl up in a ball somewhere. I assumed my professional persona and put my grief aside for my working hours. I would have all the emotions normal to my working environment. When I left work something would remind me that my father was dead. The old "nothing will be the same" voice would start up and instantly I would become dispirited and gloomy again.

Try to remember a time when you were feeling exceptionally happy and lighthearted, and you were with a friend who had suffered a loss. You put your gaiety on hold and became sympathetic and caring. We have all done it. In childhood, we were usually discouraged from feeling our feelings in the moment, so some psychotherapeutic models of the past twenty years have presented the opposite. Let it all hang out. Perhaps now we can let the pendulum center back into the middle and express our feelings when it is safe in the moment and save them for later when it is not.

This week, practice putting your less intense feelings on hold to experience later. A minor aggravation or irritation, a small sadness, would be a good starting point. Notice if you are consciously acting, holding the thought of your original emotion under the pretense of another. That isn't what I mean. See if you can actually step into another role in your repertoire that doesn't even remember the negative emotion.

Think of it this way. The actors in a soap opera are very unconvincing to me. They seem like people who can't forget for a minute that they are acting. A really good actress, Meryl Streep for example, makes me forget for two hours that I am watching actors. What is going on in the movie seems real.

A friend of mine was giving a party and her husband said something to her in front of their friends that she thought demeaning. She pretended to have a good time until the party was over and then gave him heck. She had allowed a careless remark to spoil her evening. I'm sure that has happened to all of us. If she had been able to move completely back into her party hostess role and enjoy herself, without rerunning the remark and nursing the hurt feelings underneath, she could have had a good time. Then when she brought it up later, it probably could have been clarified quite quickly. Her husband loves her dearly and had just been momentarily unconscious. It happens to the best of us, especially in party situations.

Often, when we nurse our hurt feelings in this way, it is for a purpose. We have the mistaken idea that we can change other people if only they see how much they have hurt us. Or we have the fear that if we don't show them our pain, they will do the same thing again, or worse. We are hanging on to our negative emotions in order to manipulate others. It doesn't work. So many of our behaviors don't work, and yet we refuse to give them up.

My first marriage was my schoolroom in this regard. I tried to manipulate that man to get my needs met every way I could think of for seventeen years. It *never* worked and I have to tell you I was infinitely creative. I finally had an Aha! experience when I realized that he was doing what was right for him and I had to do what was right for me. I made up my mind to always remember that I can't change anyone but me. So there was no longer any need to hang on to my pain to influence others. I can just go ahead and work on it myself and get over it sooner and get back to feeling good. What a relief!

Choices

Here are some of our choices around feelings:

✳ We can choose what we are feeling.

✳ We can choose to put our feelings on hold until we are safe.

✳ We can choose to work old pain out of our bodies by using all the incidents in our daily life that trigger the past pain for us.

✳ We can choose to use our body sensations to work through pain.

✳ We can stop deadening ourselves by repressing our feelings, and own them instead.

✳ We can stop using our feelings to manipulate others.

✳ We can explore the wonderful sensations that come from the free expression of joy and grief and all the other unlimited emotions that enrich our lives.

✳ We can acknowledge that we create all of our feelings, good and bad. No one does it to us.

✳ We can celebrate all of the choices we have around feelings.

Explorations for the Week

✳ Act out your emotions.

✳ Explore some of the above choices in your life.

✳ Get to know and appreciate your inner witness.

✳ Write three emotions you don't like to feel.

✳ Write three emotions you are uncomfortable seeing others express.

✳ Acknowledge all the ways you use your feelings to punish and manipulate others.

✳   Remember a time when you expressed what you were feeling and the situation had a happy ending.

✳   Remember a time when you did not express your feelings and it worked for you in that situation.

Resource List

 Crum, Thomas F. *The Magic of Conflict*. New York: Touchstone Books/Simon & Schuster, 1987.

Chapter Eight

LET'S GET PHYSICAL

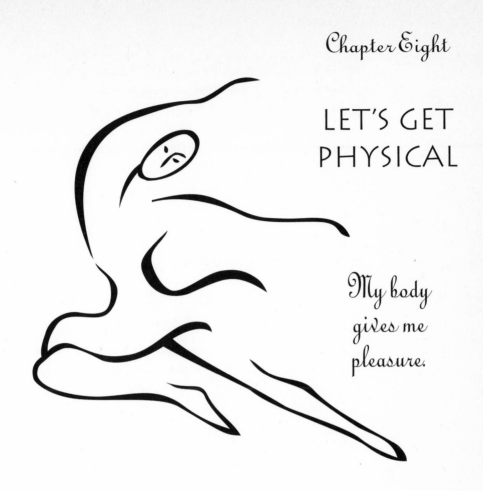

My body gives me pleasure.

When I ask my clients what it is that brings them pleasure in their bodies, I have become used to their startled reaction. Pain they know all about. Pleasure they're not sure of. They think for a while and then smile and say, "Sex" as if that must be the answer I am looking for. I remind them of the pleasure of having their skin stroked by a partner or by soft clothing, or the pleasure of lying in the sun in a garden on a spring day. "Yes, of course," they say, "I had forgotten that."

They have forgotten because they aren't usually present within their skin to experience any sensation. To be truly present with our bodies is to be ready and willing to experience totally, with all of our senses, and without comparisons. It is a left-brain tendency to pull ourselves out of an experience in order to compare it with another. To our sensation-seeking right brain, there never was another experience just like this one and never will be. This is complete and this is enough.

When were you last fully present to feel some of the following experiences:

A long, hot, sweet-smelling bath.

Massaging your body with lotion or oil.

The sun shining on your bare skin.

A warm wind or rain touching your skin.

The smell of flowers or wood smoke or new-mown grass.

The sounds of good music.

The warmth of a wood fire, crackling, dancing, and glowing.

The sensual pleasure of tasting a wonderful meal.

The freedom of walking under the stars on a warm night.

Moving through water.

Dancing.

Laughing joyfully with your whole body.

Singing.

Stretching languorously.

Making love.

Yelling.

Sucking something, our first pleasure.

Running.

Exercising.

Moving in a full range of motion.

Spinning like a child until you lose your balance.

Skipping and jumping.

Climbing a tree and sitting in it.

Walking out in nature after a rain.

Planting things in a garden.

Stroking someone.

Cuddling with someone you love.

Touching an object that was made with love.

Bringing yourself to orgasm.

Smiling with your whole body.

Hugging a friend.

Petting an animal.

Playing with a child.

Hugging a tree.

Lying on the grass watching clouds pass by.

What did I leave out? What are your own special pleasures?

This week will be an adventure into the seeking out of our pleasures. We will find whatever gives us the sensation of total delight and completeness. When we are in a state of sensory pleasure it feels as if we would be content to continue forever, and yet gradually, in our own time, we become complete with it, and move on to something else with no sense of loss.

Notice your reaction to becoming more aware of pleasure. Are you impatient? Who has time for that kind of thing? Do you feel guilty? Does the voice of duty say you are supposed to work, or bring pleasure to others, but not to yourself? Does your pleasure consist solely of getting *out* of your body—reading, watching television? Even listening to music can be an out-of-body experience if you have to sit still in a hard chair and restrict your aliveness in order to hear it. I can't listen to music any more without moving. I used to sit in a row at the symphony listening with my ears and my mind, but now I need to listen with my whole body. Thank goodness for CDs.

Reclaiming Sensuality

What does the word *sensual* mean to you? It is very different from sexual, isn't it? Picture in your imagination a woman dancing alone in a sunny meadow or a cat stretching on a windowsill. Cats are so perfectly present in their bodies in every moment. Just watching a cat stretch and roll and play makes me want to get down on the floor and join in.

Many of us lost touch with sensuality at an early age. It is a quality that has long been regarded as dangerous, even sinful. Taking pleasure in our own senses, especially touch, has been looked on with disapproval, especially for women. This is a country founded on puritanical roots, after all. Let's free ourselves of those old restrictions and move joyfully into the realm of the senses.

Explore each of your senses in a way that makes you feel completely present in your body. Using your soft gaze, look at someone or something you love as if you were caressing them. Looking at a person in this way is like discovering them all over again. Allow your eyes to wander over a beautiful plant or a hand-crafted object. Then look at yourself this way in the mirror, as if you had been blind and just regained your sight.

If you want to try something really extraordinary, blindfold yourself for half an hour and wander through your house or garden, noticing how your other senses become more alive. When you take off the blindfold you will see the beauty around you with new eyes. Just looking at the way the sun beams in the window, casting shadows on the walls, can fill you with a sense of the beauty and wonder of life.

Now try sound. Listen to music with your whole body. Do nothing else. Just feel the music flow through you.

Now get lost in your sense of smell. Fill the house with incense or cinnamon or perfume or flowers. I have planted my garden full of fragrant flowers, and whenever I can, I bring in enough to make the whole house smell. Jasmine by the side of my bed has woken me up in the middle of the night with its intensity. I lie there and float in the smell and it drifts through my dreams. No wonder perfume was considered an aphrodisiac. Right now the mimosa trees are in bloom and I have branches from them in every room.

Dedicate an entire evening to taste. Taste all the different flavors you have in the house as if experiencing each one for the first time. Let different tastes melt on your tongue—a kiwi, vanilla, honey, vinegar, some salt.

The last is my favorite, the sense of touch. Touch everything that gives you pleasure. Touch objects with your eyes shut and sense what you can from connecting surface to surface. We can survive the loss of all of our other senses, but not the sense of touch. Without sufficient touching, babies will die or fail to grow. How many of us actually get all the touching and stroking we need to feed us emotionally? Touch can heal so many of our ills. It is far better than any medicine.

Touch your face as if you were learning to recognize it in the dark. With gentle hands, feel every part of it, every nook and cranny. Do you think you could recognize your loved ones by touch alone? Get out a sweet-smelling lotion and stroke it into your skin, or take a hot bath and brush your body gently from head to toe as if you were preparing yourself for an initiation.

May I Have This Dance

Dancing is such a natural, wonderful expression of sensual joy in the moment. Joyful children dance and sing without inhibition. Then a time comes when self-consciousness sets in. We start to look at ourselves from the outside and we lose our spontaneity. As we grow up, our dancing becomes choreographed and formal, and it becomes important to do it right. Then we train our bodies to move only in the ways that are acceptable to our peers in the style of the moment. Let's forget all that and remember how to move freely for the pure joy of it.

Since many of us are threatened by the whole idea of dancing, even alone in our own space, we will start with something wonderful and easy. First, erase all images of Ginger Rogers or *Swan Lake* from your mind. We are going to redefine the word dance as any movement that gives us pleasure. That eliminates success and failure. Anyone can apply. No previous training required.

Be alone in a room with some free floor space and play some music you love. Play it *really loud*. This is important. Use headphones if you have to, but it is so much better without them. Lie on the floor in a comfortable position with your arms on the floor beside you and allow the vibration of the music to flow through you. It is an incredible experience. The drums will be playing one part of you, the flutes another. Soon your every cell will feel as if it is dancing. The music will be playing *you*.

Experiment until you find the right music. Classical music with full orchestra is perfect. Vangelis is great. Try *Heaven and Hell* or *Chariots of Fire*. If you have *The Planets* by Holst, play *Mars* when you are tired or depressed and *Venus* when you are wired. Ballets are better than opera for this. Music can change any mood in a moment. Great music affects us deeply on a cellular level. You are probably aware that different kinds of music have different effects, so for this experiment, allow your cells to choose for you.

The second time you experiment with this exercise, allow the music to move you in very small ways. Let your muscles contract and relax to the music wherever you feel it in your body. You may find you have muscles you were never aware of before. The music can persuade tight muscles to let go. Gradually move more and more until you are actually rolling around on the floor like a happy baby—stretching, reaching, rolling, curling, and stroking. Move in circles. See if you can make every joint in your body move in a circle. Circular movements are so healing to the body.

Touch yourself as you move. Some of us never touch ourselves at all except in the shower. Bring your hands alive with sensing and curiosity, and stroke yourself as you roll around. Doesn't your skin feel good? That is real sensuality—the good feelings your senses bring you. Smell your own special smell. Taste yourself. Have you ever noticed how children suck their arms and their knees as well as their fingers and thumbs. When your inner critic tells you to get up off the floor and behave like a lady, ask it politely to wait outside the door until you are finished. This is your time to play.

We are creatures. We have bodies. Our minds and our intellects would have us forget that, but our senses *long* for us to remember it. Maybe if we remember how we taste, we won't run to the refrigerator for comfort. Instead of a Ding-dong™ or a cupcake when you are feeling unloved, suck your thumb or the back of your hand. That always wakes me up to which part of me is upset. It is usually one of my inner children that needs some comforting.

Our bodies *can* be the chief source of comfort in our lives. No one else knows us like our bodies. No one else is always there for us, no matter how much they love us. People leave, people die. Take your pleasure and your comfort from your own body. Don't worry if it isn't the size or shape you would like. The pleasures of the senses are not limited to a certain weight or appearance, thank goodness. If you allow your body to please you, and live inside it more, it will adjust to its own healthy shape.

There was a time when I resented the way my skin was changing as I got older, and then I had a wonderful experience in the shower one day. I was feeling low-energy and disconnected. I looked down at my arm and suddenly I really saw myself. Isn't it amazing how you can have a shower every day for months without really seeing yourself? I saw

> That is real sensuality—the good feelings your senses bring you.

My body
and my senses
are always
there in the
moment,
available to be
tuned into
and to
bring me back
to the
magnificent
present.

my skin, the microscopic creases in it that lead from one tiny hair to another. The way it sparkled with the water droplets in thousands of rainbows. I suddenly realized for the first time that I was waterproof! The water pooled up on my skin as if I had been Scotchguarded™. What a miracle! I felt as if I had been touched by the Divine. Then it was so idiotic I laughed until my belly hurt. For the rest of the week, whenever I had a problem I would think, "I can handle this, I'm waterproof."

My mind can always find a problem to brood over if I allow it. It is endlessly inventive. My body and my senses are always there in the moment, available to be tuned into and to bring me back to the magnificent present.

Sexuality

Sex in this culture is such a commodity. Sexuality is a hard subject to approach. For most of my clients with severe pain, it turned out that their sexual experiences in the past or present were an important component of that pain. Women throughout the ages have endured so much emotional and physical pain in order to gratify their own and others' sexual urges. We have to recognize that we carry the resonance of our heritage from centuries of abuse and bondage.

We also feel, on some deep level, all of the abuse being inflicted on women right now, all over the world. We can deny this connection all we want. We can feel safe within our own relationships, but the fact is that women are not yet safe in this culture. In most places, we cannot walk alone at night. We are often not safe in our own homes. This is the undercurrent that stirs deep and dark beneath all our fears of our honest expression of our sexuality.

When women talk together openly, it seems that every woman over the age of thirty is willing to admit to some difficulties with her own sexuality. Either we have no partner, or we have the wrong partner, or we have the right partner but the wrong technique, or we have no time, or we are too stressed out. The list goes on.

During our lifetimes, there has been such change in the traditional roles in this area of life. Yet healthy sexuality can be a way of expressing every changing face of union, from an ecstatically spiritual blending with the divine to a deep exploration of our creaturehood. Sexual energy is one of the most powerful, universal energies we deal with in our lifetime. Keeping it repressed costs us more than we realize. We use up so much energy in burying our sexual feelings that we cause our bodies to stiffen up and start dying. My intuition is that in order to start to heal ourselves and others, we have to honor our own sexuality first.

Most of us were taught as young girls to cut off both sensuality and sexuality until Prince Charming arrived and then everything would be splendid. It wasn't. Then came the sexual revolution and women were acknowledged to have sexual needs equal to men's—equal rights to orgasm. For most women that didn't work either.

Most women have needs for emotional bonding and a sense of security before their sexuality can be fully expressed with another person. We have to reclaim our own sexual bodies and learn to pleasure ourselves first. When we can explore and delight in our sexuality alone, to the point of orgasm, then we can be truly safe. Orgasm is good for our bodies. It enhances the immune system. If we can give ourselves that gift joyfully, we can move into choice in the area of relationship.

Many women I know have made the choice to live without a partner of either sex. They feel the need to pursue their spiritual path through life basically alone, with the love and support of their friends. This is a perfectly valid choice and certainly a common one through history. It is also a fact that women live longer than men and many women are alone through no choice of their own. Whether or not we choose the

When we can explore and delight in our sexuality alone, to the point of orgasm, then we can be truly safe.

path of relationship is not the issue. The issue is that if we hold the key to our own sexuality, then we can keep ourselves healthy in the moment by giving *ourselves* the gift of orgasm.

Pelvic Circles

The way we have most effectively controlled our sexuality is by holding the pelvis rigid. By doing this, we create an energy blockage in the whole area of the genitals and lower back so that we will not have to feel the feelings that arise there. Any time we hold any part of our body rigid we are affecting our whole lives. Rigidity spreads.

If I hold my pelvis stiff, I cannot walk freely because my hips can't rotate, and then my arms don't swing loosely so my shoulders get tight. Lower back pain is often related to a chronically tight pelvic area. Hip and knee problems develop from the same cause. If you don't give a hoot about orgasm, never had it, never want it, then do this exercise for the health of the rest of your body.

✳   Lie on your back with your knees up.

✳   Repeat each movement at least ten times, slowly, gently, and lovingly. Be fully present.

✳   Imagine the clock face on your body as you did in the rocking breath. Twelve is at your heart, six at your knees, three is at your left hip and nine at your right hip. The center of the clock is your tailbone touching the floor.

✳   Start rocking your pelvis slowly from twelve to six and back. This is a small, soft movement. Your bottom does not pick up off the floor.

✳   Now rock from three to nine and back. Don't flop your knees from side to side. The movement is in your pelvis.

✳   Now go around the clock in a circle from twelve to three to six to nine to twelve. Make your circle as round as possible. If you go slowly enough, you will notice the places where your circle is not round.

✳ Reverse the circle. Remember to move gently and sensually.

Gradually, as you practice this movement every day, you can add more numbers to your clock and fine tune your awareness of where your pelvis is in the circle. The muscles that move the pelvis are among the strongest in the body and freeing them up to move will affect every movement you make. You can also practice these pelvic circles while sitting and standing. When done standing, they are reminiscent of belly dancing or the Hawaiian hula.

After you practice pelvic circles every day for a while, you will probably notice that you are feeling more sensual. You may start to be more aware of your genital area. You may feel the flow of energy from your sexual center for the first time. Many of my clients were afraid of this feeling. They were afraid they would be compelled to do something they would be ashamed of, like going to a bar and picking up a stranger.

Getting in touch with our own flow of sexuality doesn't make us suddenly out of control. Opening up to the experience of our feelings doesn't mean we need to express those feelings inappropriately. We can always learn to bring ourselves to orgasm with a little experimenting and practice.

Be gentle with yourself. Seek out the pleasure centers of your own body. Men have limited their erogenous zones to a small area, but for women, our whole body can be an erogenous zone. There are sex manuals for women to learn from, but if you give yourself the freedom to explore, you probably won't need them. Make up a fantasy in your imagination. You are unlimited. You can create anything that pleases you.

Women often turn to vibrators to pleasure themselves, but I have found that vibrators don't work for me. I think they are too mechanistic and lead to multiple, shallow sensations rather than a full orgasmic release. Many women have told me that they need a male to come to orgasm because they like the feeling of penetration. I thought so too until I learned the next exercise.

You are unlimited. You can create anything that pleases you.

Lie down with your knees up the same as before, and experiment with contracting all of the muscles of the pelvic floor. You will be tightening everything as if you needed to go to the bathroom and you couldn't find one. Contract and relax at least twenty times.

Next, try to isolate the muscles of your vagina from those in your buttocks. You will probably not succeed completely at first. Do the best you can. A way to practice this is to start and stop the flow of urine next time you go to the bathroom.

When you have the control of the muscles in the vagina isolated, think of the opening of the vagina as the first floor in a seven-story building and gradually tighten up on each floor as you climb up to the top. Some deep, internal belly muscles will be activated. Tighten gradually and relax gradually—up and down as if you were riding an escalator in the building. Make sure the muscles in your buttocks are as relaxed as possible.

This exercise approximates the feelings of penetration and has enormous benefits. It will encourage orgasm if you are pleasuring yourself. It will make you a more exciting lover. It will help you to avoid the problems of collapsing organs later in life, and it will aid in preventing you from having problems with incontinence.

The whole media marketing program pushing diapers for women makes me angry. This is not a natural part of aging. Don't buy into it. Lack of movement and lack of stimulation for the muscles of the pelvic floor lead to incontinence, and both can be corrected. We can make internal changes in our muscle tone instead of relying on external props. I taught a friend of mine to do these exercises in one session and she called later and said she had been practicing in the car and had spontaneous orgasms all the way home. Time for a drive?

If you are embarrassed to even think of experimenting with your own sexuality, ask the shy teenager or the disapproving parent within you to wait outside the door for a while and just try it. All of this is normal behavior for adult women and is nothing to be ashamed of. It is *your* body. Learn to enjoy it

completely while alone and you may choose to share that pleasure with a partner at some point in time when you are ready.
If you have a partner, don't feel guilty for experimenting alone.
You aren't being disloyal. You are learning something that will
ultimately benefit you both.

Sexuality After Menopause

Isn't it funny that you couldn't say the word "menopause" in
polite company fifteen years ago and now we never stop hearing about it. Many of my post-menopausal clients who are
alone put sex out of their minds and bodies with relief, leaving
"all that" behind them. If this applies to you, you may not have
even read parts of this chapter, thinking you don't need it.

Turning off our sexuality is not good for the body. The hormonal system is one of our "use it or lose it" systems, and the
hormones we manufacture when we are feeling sexual benefit
our bodies in many ways. Osteoporosis is endemic in this culture among older women, and the activity of our hormonal
system vitally affects the health of our bones.

It is sometimes difficult to begin your sexual life anew when
you have given it up so completely. Start out by allowing yourself some sensual experiences, memories, and thoughts. Stop
censoring yourself. Find some fiction of the exact kind of sexuality that stirs you, or make up your own fantasies.

When I have been busy on a creative project for a while, it
sometimes occurs to me that I haven't felt sexual for ages. I
think my intuition reminds me. So I give myself a sensual
evening, a date with myself—music, bubble bath, wine, and
everything to set the mood. A part of me seems to sigh and say,
"Thank goodness. I thought you had forgotten me."

I will finish this chapter with a Feldenkrais story. In my
training we loved these stories. My master teacher was giving a
demonstration of Feldenkrais work in front of a group of doc-
tors. The client was an elderly woman who was in extreme

pain with her back and very stiff all over. He started to work with her, gently moving her as far as her restrictions would allow. As he got closer to her pelvic area, she stiffened up even more and started to clench her fists. Finally, as he rocked her pelvis gently, she started pounding the table and yelling, "No!" She was as surprised as he at this reaction.

What came to her awareness was that she was terribly angry with her husband, who had died six months before. They had enjoyed loving sexual relations right up until his death and she had tried to deny her loss by stiffening up entirely. After the session her pain was gone and she was able to move through her anger and grief and get on with her life.

Explorations for the Week

* This week, choose your own homework from all the material in the chapter. Ease in slowly, be kind to yourself, love yourself, and keep a sense of fun.

Resource List

Louden, Jennifer. *The Women's Comfort Book*. San Francisco: HarperCollins Publishers, 1992.

Roth, Gabriella. *The Wave—Intuitive Dance Video*. 1-800-76RAVEN. (Wonderful for dancing alone.)

Conger, Nancy. *Sensuous Living*. St. Paul: Llewellyn Publications, 1996.

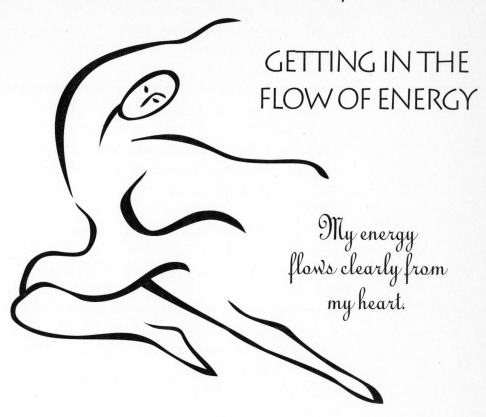

Chapter Nine

GETTING IN THE FLOW OF ENERGY

My energy flows clearly from my heart.

Like all living things, we are all unique patterns of energy that have danced their way into matter. We float in an endless field of energy that most of us cannot see with our outer eyes. We have luminous, bright-colored clouds of energy all around us, and our energy fields embrace each other long before our bodies ever connect. Science is finally measuring and photographing these fields so that they can be proven to the entire satisfaction of the left brain. Our right brains see, feel and know information intuitively, without words, and our left brains mock anything that cannot be explained and measured. This split is healed only when we invent better tools to measure what cannot be seen. It has happened throughout history. People in the West, who honor the left brain above everything, didn't believe the world was round until they proved it, didn't believe in germs, didn't believe in Evolution.

Now there is a new paradigm shift occurring. The old Newtonian world view has changed to the new view of the Quantum universe. The Newtonian way of looking at things was simple. It was a mechanistic world view. We are all separate and when we do things to each other we set up a chain of reactions, like billiard balls colliding.

The new ideas of Quantum Physics say the same as mystics have claimed since recorded time began. We are all one. I don't have to collide with you to affect your life. I can affect you merely by being in your energy field, or even by living my own life in my own way. The Chaos theory says that a butterfly fluttering in China can create a pattern that may become an electrical storm in New England. We are discovering anew, on the leading edge of thought, how connected we all are. The flow of energy is the magical medium of connection.

Remember a situation you were observing, not participating in. You could have been at an airport or in a crowded room and someone you could see was behaving in a way that either touched your heart or made you angry. Without any personal involvement, you have been affected. Are you separate from that event now that it has touched you?

When I think of images that have touched millions of people deeply and initiated great change, there are two that come instantly to mind. The picture of the little Vietnamese girl running with her clothes burned off from napalm was seared into my memory and seemed to be an important turning point in public opinion about the Vietnam war. The first pictures of the Earth sent back from outer space changed forever the way many people connected with their planet. In the same way, a movie or play or novel can deeply affect the way we see our world. Remember a movie you saw recently that changed the way you thought or felt about some issue.

Now remember an occasion when you saw a person for the first time and felt immediate attraction or repulsion. What were you responding to? Was it body language? Was it their resemblance to someone in your memory banks? Or was it the subtle energy field, called the aura, that emanates from all of us? We all read these fields unconsciously as we go through our day, but some people read them more clearly and are less easily fooled than others. You *can* learn to read these energy fields consciously.

Think of an adjective to describe *yourself* as you meet someone for the first time. How would a person who never saw you before describe you in one word—shy, arrogant, controlling, beautiful, kind, overbearing, depressed? Would they see the real you in that description or are you projecting a convincing image? Most of us would like to give the impression that we have our act together, that we have all our ducks in a row.

My brother, Derek, calls some people he meets Posers, meaning they aren't real; they are hiding behind an act. Are you a Poser or do you allow who you are and what you are feeling in the moment to show? Do you think you can detect a Poser? When you improve on your natural ability to read the energy fields of others, they will not be able to fool you. You will know when someone is angry, and whether that anger is their habitual state or just a fleeting emotion. You will know when someone is feeling truly happy and powerful, or just covering up inner sadness or fear with a cheerful facade.

Whenever we are false, other people know it on some level of awareness, if not consciously. Remember a time when you were with someone who was putting on an act. We can either play along with the act ourselves or we can cut right through it by being clear and honest. It seems to me that there is a lot less pretense now than when I was a child. It was always very confusing to me when grown-ups said one thing and I could see that they were feeling the opposite.

Do *you* remember the honesty and clarity you had as a child? Can you imagine a world in which no one could lie and get away with it? It is my belief that we already live in that world but, as in the story of the Emperor's New Clothes, no one wants to be the first to acknowledge it. Our energy fields always reveal exactly who we are and how we are feeling; they give us away.

Personal Energy Fields

Our energy field extends out around us and becomes subtler and subtler, like mist. Close to the body, it has various colors that indicate our state of mind. Inside the body, which is the denser part of our beingness, the energy runs most powerfully on certain meridians or pathways. Different ancient philosophies, such as the Indian or the Chinese, have slightly different patterns of pathways. The spinal pathway has seven chakras or energy wheels at seven locations on our spine where certain different energies are expressed.

If this is all new to you, it may well sound like New Age baloney. It is actually very ancient wisdom, so bear with me. When you experience the energy running through you, you will know the truth of it. Until then it is just words.

If you have been doing the Heaven and Earth breath regularly, by now you have probably experienced the sensation of energy in your heart or moving up your spine or through your hands. People experience this sensation in various ways—as heat, light, tingling, or shaking.

When I send intense energy while doing healing work, my hands actually vibrate. Some of my clients have thought I was nervous or tired because they don't feel the flow of energy, just the shaking. Do you recall the image of heat on a road stretching into the distance on a hot day, the mirage effect? That is how it seems to me. A shimmer that can get more and more intense, leading my hands into a kind of trembling.

When you experience the energy running through you, you will know the truth of it.

Try an Experiment

To experience your own energy field, sit quietly, cross-legged or on a chair, with both feet on the ground. Close your eyes and imagine a wheel spinning like a child's toy at the level of your heart between your breasts. This is the heart chakra. It is the center of love energy and is the easiest to access at first. Bring into your mind an image of a time when you deeply loved someone or something innocent, like a child or a kitten or a flower. Feel the energy of that pure, simple feeling intensify in your heart like sunshine. Know that this feeling of love is all around us all the time, waiting for us to open our hearts to receive it.

With your imagination, turn up the volume on that feeling until you feel a physical sensation in your heart, a stirring. You may feel your heart brimming over, as if it holds enough love for the whole Universe.

It is often necessary to keep the mind focused on a simple task so it quiets down and gives you some space to experience. If your mind is busy with thoughts, concentrate on repeating the words, "I am love." Imagine that the words come out of your heart. Breathe deeply, exhale fully.

When you feel a clear energy in your heart, send it down both of your arms to your hands just by willing it to flow there. You may feel them tingle or light up in some way. Now put your hands facing each other about a foot apart and create a bridge across the space with the energy you are sending. You can feel the energy jump across the space to connect and form a circle from your heart through your hands and back again to your heart. Relax your shoulders. You don't have to force anything, just surrender and allow the energy to move through you.

When you are finished, pull the energy back from your hands to your heart, take a couple of deep breaths, and let it go. Does it feel as if you reached into a bottomless well of heart energy? Do you feel revitalized and optimistic?

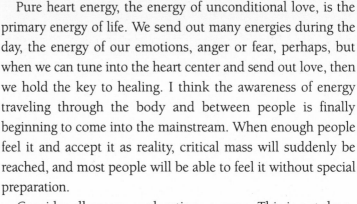

Pure heart energy, the energy of unconditional love, is the primary energy of life. We send out many energies during the day, the energy of our emotions, anger or fear, perhaps, but when we can tune into the heart center and send out love, then we hold the key to healing. I think the awareness of energy traveling through the body and between people is finally beginning to come into the mainstream. When enough people feel it and accept it as reality, critical mass will suddenly be reached, and most people will be able to feel it without special preparation.

Consider all energy explorations a game. This is not drop-dead serious. Too much effort makes it harder to learn. Take it lightly. Many people think that if they imagine something, it is not real. The fact is that everything we create is created first in the imagination and then in reality. By opening to the possibility of feeling our energy moving through us, we eventually enable ourselves to actually feel it. Sometimes we have to tune in to that particular channel on our receivers for a while before the message comes through.

It is much easier to learn to move energy from a person who does it well and can induct you with their presence, but with patience and trust you can also learn alone. Don't allow yourself to feel like a failure over this. Thinking that you can't do it is the fastest way to block energy flow. Given time and intention, anyone can experience energy.

Have you tried looking at those computer-generated 3D pictures that have been so popular? You look and look and when you finally give up looking you can see. At a workshop I went to, some of us saw the wonderful, deep, inner image instantly. Most people saw it after some practice, and some people got frustrated and angry and couldn't see it until they gave up trying hours later. What we shared was our amazement that the picture was so completely invisible to regular sight and yet so clear when looked at in the right way. It is the same with energy.

People have difficulty feeling something as obvious as their own pulse at first. Think of how many substances are flowing around and through our bodies all the time outside of our conscious awareness—blood, lymph, cerebrospinal fluid, hormones, etc. Is it so hard to believe that energy does the same thing? It is like our own personal electrical system. It can't be seen directly, but it's effects can surely be felt with a little practice. When I work with groups of beginners and they start to feel the flow, there is always such a sense of joy, even relief. People realize they have been missing an important element of their lives.

Feeling our energy consciously is a quantum leap on the road to home. Home is the place where we remember we are immortal, boundless, limitless, and able to live our lives with a sense of peace and wonder. We are all so much bigger than our day-to-day struggles, but we get caught up in our dramas and forget. Practice this exercise of sitting and growing your awareness of pure heart energy as often as you can.

This universal love energy that connects all things is not a personal love, it is an unconditional love, and it is our birthright. A few people throughout the ages have always been able to feel it. They are the ones we have called mystics. Now the ability is spreading so that we can all have access to this unconditional love state whenever we choose.

Frequent practice really helps. Many people would like to learn to see auras and seem to expect to see clear rainbows of color with their physical eyes. I have found that feeling energy through the heart center is the best and safest road for most of us. There is less danger of being caught in ego power states. Seeing auras is much easier, if you want to, after you have felt heart energy run through your own body.

> Home is the place where we remember we are immortal, boundless, limitless, and able to live our lives with a sense of peace and wonder.

The Chakra System

The most widely accepted energy system is the Spinal Pathway with the seven spinning chakras. It is an ancient system from the Vedic texts of India. Here is a highly simplified explanation.

There are many books available that deal more completely with the various chakra systems. My intention is to give you enough of a structure so that you can more easily experience the energy for yourself.

Within the Christian tradition, Jesus worked extensively with energy. He said, "Anything that I can do, you can also do and greater." The laying-on of hands that Jesus did was simply the transmission of healing energy. Many nuns and nursing sisters are using the same techniques today. Therapeutic touch is one of the names given to this kind of healing.

✳   The first chakra is at the base of the spine and connects us to the earth, to the physical plane. Do you know someone who has this energy in abundance? They will seem very grounded, very down-to-earth, very practical. The color is red. When you do the Heaven and Earth breath, this chakra is awakened by the earth energy you pull up your spine. This chakra is involved whenever we have issues with our security. People who are unawakened in this chakra are likely to be very spacey and unrealistic; they don't seem at all sure that they want to be here on the Earth in a body.

✳   The second chakra is just above your pubic bone and is the sexual and creative chakra. Think of someone you know who is sensual, not overtly sexy since that is usually an act, but someone who enjoys the whole world of touch. This color is orange.

You will feel this chakra ignite when you are attracted to someone sexually. Have you ever been having an ordinary conversation with someone and suddenly a sexual spark lights up between you from a look, a touch, a certain word? That is your second chakra reminding you that you are a sexual being. You don't have to act on it, just enjoy the reminder. Since this chakra covers the whole world of creativity as well as sexual creativity, you may find during periods when you are without a love partner that you are suddenly creative in many other ways.

❋ The third chakra is above your navel and is the emotional chakra. Do you know anyone who can express her feelings honestly in the moment and then move right back to peace and joy? This color is yellow. This chakra is highly volatile and its desires also don't have to be acted upon. Just notice which emotion is being played out and appreciate it. A person who has a lot of energy centered on their emotional chakra often tends to be involved in power struggles. Our emotions can be easily used to control others.

❋ The fourth chakra is the heart, the love center. My friend, Lilli, personifies this one for me. She takes in lost people the way other women take in lost cats and lovingly sets them on their feet again. This color is green. This is the center for all kinds of love, including the highest—unconditional love.

   Few people can manifest this kind of love that sees all and expects nothing, and needs nothing in return. It is the love our Higher Self has for us. This chakra is the center of our energy system and the most in need of awakening right now. Whenever you are in doubt about anything in your life, bring your awareness back to the heart center and rest there. This is where the energy of the earth and the energy of Spirit are equally at home and can mix to bring balance to our lives.

Whenever you are in doubt about anything in your life, bring your awareness back to the heart center and rest there.

❋ The next chakra point, located between the heart and the throat, has no number because it is not mentioned in the old systems. Brugh Joy calls it the mid-chest chakra. It is an energy point that has to do with regeneration and rejuvenation. We are developing and changing as spiritual beings all the time, you could say evolving, and it is very important to open to and appreciate this chakra.

❋ The fifth chakra, at the throat, is the energy of true and wise speech and of verbal creativity. Think of someone you know who always says the magical words that heal your heart. I have had to work hard on this one. I often spoke in haste and repented at leisure. This color is blue. If your sexual or emotional chakras are over-active, you can set the intention to balance the energy up to this chakra and you will have a burst of creativity of some kind.

❋ The sixth chakra is at the third eye between the eyebrows and has two energies, that of the mind and that of the inner wisdom. Do you know anyone who lets their intuition guide their life, listening to the voice of inner wisdom on all decisions? Your mind can very easily lead you astray since it is often led by the ego, but your Inner Wisdom never will. This color is purple. I usually finish my meditation by connecting the energy of my heart center with this chakra, seeking to see clearly from my heart and my intuition.

❋ The seventh chakra is at the crown of the head and is the energy of spirit. This is where we connect with Source and Home, our limitless self. This color is clear bright light.

Your mind can very easily lead you astray since it is often led by the ego, but your Inner Wisdom never will.

The ideal is to have the energy running through all the chakras in a perfect balance for you on your particular life path. For instance, at some points in our lives, and even some points in our monthly cycles, the energy in the sexual center will be more pronounced, other times less so. We usually feel more energy at the emotional center when we have change and disturbance in our lives.

The important thing is to appreciate the flow of energy, not allowing it to get stuck at any one spot. We will know when we are blocked because, like a stuck record, we will keep repeating the same thoughts over and over, thoughts of need or lack or problems. Our bodies will also reveal energy blocks by becoming stiff or unresponsive or painful. At those moments, breathe deeply or dance or do the Heaven and Earth breath to get the energy flowing again.

We do not actually create energy ourselves, although it often seems as if we do. We merely channel the energy that is all around us all the time. Like electricity, no one knows exactly how it works. We take in pure energy from the field around us and by tuning into our thoughts and feelings it can come out through us as love, fear, anger, despair, hope, joy, or a million other patterns. It is the same energy. What we create with it is our choice. Just as we can choose to use the breath and the food that we take into our bodies for playing or working or fighting or lying around.

It may sometimes seem easier to create anger or drama in order to get a stuck situation moving again, but we could just as easily choose love. What we choose to create with the energy available to us is usually the result of our own childhood learning, but we are not the victims of our past. By resting into our heart center and repeating "I am love" for as long as it takes for our energy to shift, we can choose from a mature position of feminine power.

No matter how stuck we are, we can always ask our Inner Wisdom for help in seeing the larger perspective or the perspective of the heart. We have only to be willing to give up our ego needs to be right or to be in control. That's all! No big deal!

Relating to Others with Energy

Every time we interact with someone else we are exchanging energy. If you remember that your energy field extends out from your body, it is easy to understand why you are more comfortable with some people close to you than others. The distance our field extends around us varies according to how open and expanded we feel. Sometimes when we don't feel safe, our aura becomes dense and is very close to our body. When someone approaches, we can tell in a millisecond whether this person is safe and what energy they are sending us. So much of our communication goes on energetically before we ever *say* anything.

Spend a few days noticing the quality of your energy and how you send energy to others. Check which way the energy is flowing between you. Are you expanding or contracting, giving or receiving? Do you feel fed by your interactions? Think of energy as the invisible component of support or encouragement. Who is doing the feeding, the supporting? You know how to feed someone who is joyful and you know how to steal their joy away in a moment, don't you?

Imagine doing that with a friend. She comes toward you full of joyous news and you intensify her pleasure by joining in it with her. You are feeding her joy with your energy. Now imagine saying something negative and watch her pleasure wilt away. You could say that has nothing to do with energy, that it is the words that count. So now imagine saying the right words of congratulation, but not meaning them and feeling jealousy in your heart. The words won't help. She will feel your hidden sadness and her joy will lose its luster.

Now for more practice. From a distance, watch pairs of people interacting and guess who is sending the most energy and who is receiving or resisting. When you are learning by watching others, some clues for the direction and quality of the energy are body language, facial expression, and voice animation. It is interesting to guess which quality of energy people are sending. From the mind chakra, the energy can be in the form of stimulating conversation or debate, the exchange of ideas. Even listening to someone's ideas with interest is sending energy from the sixth chakra. From the fourth chakra, the energy is always love. From the emotional chakra, we can send energy in the form of any emotion we choose. Sometimes the energy will feed people and sometimes it will deplete them.

For example, if you are being pathetic, you are unconsciously asking for a dose of energy. If your friend is a nurturer, she will provide the supportive energy for you. If your friend is not inclined to give you the energy of support, she may get irritated at your neediness and send you the energy of anger. You have still been fed with energy and you may still feel more alive than you did before. This is how children learn to attract negative attention and feed from it.

There are very few interactions in which we send and receive equally. Notice if you are always sending energy, pouring love and help into your friends' empty spaces. Many friendships are unequal in this way. In a healthy relationship we take turns, sometimes giving and sometimes receiving. Also notice when you overwhelm others with your energy. They will often physically back away. Love *or* anger can be overwhelming to many people and much of the energy we send out has demands and needs attached to it.

So few people are sending out unconditional love energy in their lives. We take the basic, unconditional love energy of the Universe and we move it through our chakra system and transform it into something less pure. In the same way, electricity can light up a concert hall or activate the electric chair. By becoming clearer and more honest to ourselves and owning our emotions, we become clearer transformers of this universal energy.

Notice that most people have set limits on what they can give or receive. Feel your own limits. Are they different with different people in your life? Energy is the same as any other gift that someone can give us. From some people we can accept a present and from some we cannot. We can also tell instantly if a gift has strings attached. What we do most of the time is to establish boundaries around ourselves so that we can feel safe. Imagine these boundaries as wooden fences.

Notice how high your fences are with certain people, and how they vary with your mood. When your fences are high and dense, notice the reaction of people around you. Watch other people's fences fluctuate. When you notice that someone's fences are up, send them a gentle blessing of pure love energy or give them an encouraging word or a touch and watch the fences disintegrate. It is a true test of the level of heart energy we send out to another when their defenses crumble and they feel safe in being vulnerable with us.

Notice also if you are willing to be vulnerable to others. We are all so afraid to risk. We censor so much. It seems to me that we often hold back on our vibrant aliveness, the intensity of love and joy we have access to feeling and sharing. This is a choice we make moment by moment to fit in with the people around us.

I remember in my family if I was happy or exuberant, my older sister would manage to punish me somehow. But if I was depressed or upset, I got a payoff of attention from my mother. So guess what I learned! I have a firm belief that our natural state is joy, and like bubbles rising in boiling water, it will emerge any time it is able to. At eighteen, I traveled six thousand miles to be alone in a new country so I could find my way back to joy. There is a driving force within all of us to be whole and to experience our feelings and our energy fields freely.

The Protective Force

When you begin to become aware of your interactions with others on an energetic level, you may notice that you feel drained and depleted after being with certain people. We all have our own store of personal energy that we create by breathing, moving, and eating. You can imagine how much this store can vary according to the depth of our breath, our eating habits, and how much moving around we do. Even if you are very active and eat wisely, your personal store of energy is finite. By tuning into the universal supply and becoming a channel of energy as you learned in the Heaven and Earth breath, you can tap into an unlimited source of energy that you can draw on at will.

There may be times when you feel unable to draw on this universal source because of the negativity of the situation you are in at the moment. To avoid becoming depleted by the negative energy of others, you can easily learn to protect and shield yourself. Following is a tool you should practice alone before you need it so that when the time comes it can be used almost instantaneously.

Imagine yourself surrounded by an egg of white light. Some people like to call this Christ energy. I call it the light of Spirit. This egg of light can protect your energy field from intrusion and keep you from harm.

A few years ago I was traveling alone in Bali and I regretted being alone. It is a Muslim country and there is no respect for single women there. I felt off-center and bothered as I got onto a truck taxi to go across the island, but the truck was full of market women so I felt safe. We drove down a dirt road deep into a beautiful old volcano and all the women got off at their village at the bottom. I was left in the back of the truck with the two men who ran the taxi, and I knew right away I was in trouble. The two men started harassing me for more money, and then they sat beside me and started touching me. I thought I was as good as dead. I was full of fear.

Then my son's face came into my mind and I suddenly remembered to surround myself with white light. I closed my eyes, pulled the energy of Spirit around me, and instantly felt more powerful. I got up and sat on the other side of the taxi and told the men loudly and firmly that they were not going to get anything more out of me. One of them came over and sat beside me and reached out toward me again. I looked him in the eye with a new feeling of safety instead of fear, and he gave a shamefaced grin and left me alone. These were simple people and they were not under the influence of drugs. I don't recommend that you test the limits of the "White Light of Protection" foolishly, but if you ever need it, you can call on it.

The Energy of Touch

Touching
someone with
energy running
through
your hands,
and with your
heart open,
is a gift
we can give
anyone,
anywhere,
anytime.

When you touch others, always be aware of how powerful touch can be. Touching someone with energy running through your hands, and with your heart open, is a gift we can give anyone, anywhere, anytime. In the medical system in this country, there is not enough credit given to the healing power of touch. If you touch someone as you would a loved child, they *will* feel better. If you touch someone without loving awareness in your hands, you can take care of their bodily needs, but they will feel isolated and invaded, like an object.

It is an inspiration to me that so many nurses are learning the various techniques of healing touch. I am in a spiritual group with many women who are nurses and they are tired of being medical technicians. They know the power of touch, energy, and words on sick people and they wish they had more time for that kind of personal involvement.

I recently asked my Inner Wisdom how people could get sick at all when we are always surrounded by healing energy. I wanted to know the purpose of a healer. The answer I got was that a healer is someone who can focus the energy and direct it. Electricity needs wires and plugs, radio waves need receivers, laser beams need some kind of focusing machine. Healing energy needs us.

Science acknowledges that electricity, radio waves, and light are around us all the time, but without focus they are not useful. We can all learn to focus healing energy. It is not difficult at all; but don't confuse healing with curing. Don't always expect your energy to make a person well. There is too much we do not yet know about why people get the illnesses they get. Sometimes the energy we send to someone who is very sick will help them to move through the dying process more easily. Let them be the judge of what they do with your gift.

Try an Experiment

At a time when your heart is closed and you have a lot on your mind, touch someone you love and notice their response. Another time, with the energy of love flowing in your heart and in your hands, touch them again in the same place without saying anything, and notice the different response. If they are caught up in their mind and closing out feeling, they may not react in an obviously different way immediately, but usually, being touched with love will bring anyone back into their body.

We hug a lot in California. A hug is a very good test of the ability to send and receive energy. You can hug ten different people and you will have ten different experiences according to how much energy they are willing to let flow between you. Have you ever hugged someone and felt as if they weren't there? It is such a blessing when family members are in the habit of hugging hello and good-bye. Both people can tell immediately, without words, how the other person is feeling. Whole body contact reveals so much. The energy exchange is so direct.

Communicating with Energy

I believe the only useful way to communicate deeply on matters of importance is heart to heart with energies open and flowing. Anything less will result in some level of misunderstanding. Since we all come from our own experience and our own family background, we just *think* we are speaking the same language. It is an illusion. Everyone has a different intonation of meaning for the words, the tone of voice, the intensity, and the context. It is actually a miracle that we can communicate at all. It is only because we are picking up clues from our intuition and energy fields that we understand as well as we do.

Notice how clear you can be when you are fully present, speaking from your heart to someone who is willing to be present in listening. Many women complain that their men don't listen to them. The fact is that women often talk before making sure the receiver is tuned in to their station.

Men cannot do two things at once as well as women because of the physical organization of their brains, so first you have to get the man's full attention. Then find out if he is willing to receive your communication. That will indicate that his heart is open to you to some degree. Then say what you need to say clearly from your heart. Otherwise you may as well talk to the wall. I know this is a long process and often seems bothersome, but if you need to be truly *heard* about something important, it is worth making the effort.

You probably already know that women have the opposite problem, of course. We are so busy doing four things at once that we sometimes hear the words of the communication and miss the music, the true meaning. We also have to be willing to put everything else on hold and listen with our hearts whenever it is necessary. Most of the women in the groups I have been in agree that to have someone listen to them with complete attention and acceptance is the most healing thing in the world. We don't need most of the advice we are given; we just need to be heard.

I have set the intention to speak directly from my heart, my emotions, or my wisdom centers, and my belly has become my internal feedback device. Now I get an unpleasant physical sensation in my belly and my legs whenever I use words to justify or blame or gossip. I think many women learned to use words as their chief defense in growing up, as I did, but now that we are grown, it is safe to let that defense go.

When my mind is in charge of my mouth, I have learned to expect miscommunication because my mind is clever, has it's own agenda, and often forgets how powerfully destructive words can be. I try to remember to send energy from my heart up to my throat whenever I speak to someone vulnerable or someone who doesn't know me well. I blame my sometimes tactless tongue on being an Aries. I do see value in being simple and direct, but I have to make sure my heart is in the right place and I am sending out love energy.

Energy is such a fascinating subject for me. I just love it, and this is merely a beginning of the exploration. I hope you have experienced enough of the actual flow of energy to acknowledge its reality. By keeping this awareness in the back of your mind, you will learn how to relate better to your own energy patterns and cycles, as well as to others.

Remember that we are never the same. In every moment we have a different expression of our energy field. We are constantly changing like a beautiful kaleidoscope. Wanting the safety of the known, we try to stop our own flow through our lives, and that is where we block our natural spontaneity and joy. Let yourself flow, with the ups and downs, the rhythms, the cycles, the seasons, the tides of your emotions, your needs and desires.

Moshe Feldenkrais said it is desire that drives us through our lives. Our needs are basic to all of us—food, shelter, clothing, etc. Our desires are unique to each one of us, and it is the drive to satisfy these desires that causes us to move and expand and grow. Without desire we would be like stagnant ponds. Desire pulls energy in from the Universe for creation. That is the pattern of a fulfilled life: curiosity and desire pulling in healing, love, and wisdom energy for creativity and expansion. If we settle for anything less than that we are selling ourselves short.

Explorations for the Week

* Practice the sitting exercise as often as possible, pulling energy into your heart.

* Study energy flows between people.

✳   Watch interactions from a distance and practice reading which way energy is flowing.

✳   Imagine the seven chakras in your own body. Before you go to sleep at night, put your hand gently on each location and send energy from your heart to open each chakra. Ask your Inner Wisdom to balance your energies while you sleep.

✳   Experience the different energies you can send out from the different chakras. Send a friend sexual energy, joy, anger, love, and wisdom, and ask them to guess which you are sending.

✳   Practice sending energy from your heart to light up your hands, and then touch children or animals or someone who is sick.

Resource List

Joy, Brugh. *Joy's Way*. Los Angeles: J. P. Tarcher, Inc., 1978.

Redfield, James. *The Celestine Prophecy*. New York: Warner Books, 1993.

Dale, Cyndi. *New Chakra Healing*. St. Paul: Llewellyn Publications, 1996.

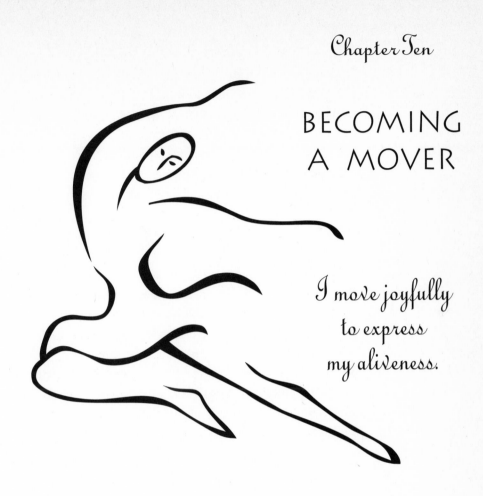

Chapter Ten

BECOMING
A MOVER

*I move joyfully
to express
my aliveness.*

Can you remember watching a healthy toddler or small child? They are never still. They run and fuss and wriggle and squirm every second they are awake. Now see if you can remember your first day of school? The school that had desks or tables where you were supposed to sit still for ages and speak only when you were told you could. How was that for you? Have you buried that memory? It was in school that we were most firmly socialized into non-movement. Sit still, sit up straight, pay attention, concentrate, no slumping, stop wriggling, no talking, no giggling, take things seriously, do it right. The only person all that control was healthy for was the teacher.

Our present educational system is simply *not* a positive environment for learning. It is no wonder that so many of us have trouble with authority figures or with learning new skills. I think it is a tribute to our in-born curiosity and desire to learn and grow that we managed to accomplish as much as we did. Imagine if we had been taught to anchor our mental activity in our bodies. Maybe we would be using a little more of our brains than the five percent we now use.

Dyslexic children have had a lot of success in learning to read by looking at letters repetitively as they bounce on a mini-trampoline. Movement can make us all learn and work better. Prove it for yourself. The next time you have to learn something new, move around a little in a way that is pleasing to you while you are learning. See if you feel more present with the learning experience. You could also try learning two verses of a poem—one while being still and the other while swinging your foot or tapping your fingers. A couple of days later, see what you retain. If you get stuck, repeat the motion you were doing while you were learning.

Needing complete stillness in order to do mental work is unnatural. I had one teacher who always said she should be able to hear a pin drop while the class was taking a test. How bizarre! Thank goodness things have changed since then. My son went to a Montessori School and it was such a pleasure to visit the classroom and see kids all over the place, working alone or cooperating on different tasks. They were all moving around naturally. I have gone to workshops and lectures with people of my own age group, and they sit on hard chairs for hours and barely move a muscle. I can't do it. I have to sit in the back or in the aisle so I can wriggle.

Learn to Wriggle

Whenever you have to stand for any length of time, waiting around or waiting in line, get used to moving your body in small ways, almost micro-movements. Travel your awareness through your body from your feet up to your head and see how many muscles you can contract and relax in such small increments that no one notices.

Try it now with your face alone. Our faces are incredibly mobile. Just one small movement can change our expression completely. First see if you can move your facial muscles so slightly that no one can tell. Now try moving as few muscles in your face as possible to change your expression. Try curious, delighted, annoyed, impatient, quizzical, amused, loving, disbelieving, disapproving, satisfied, or any one of your common expressions. I know a man who spent two years in front of a mirror learning to isolate the movements of his facial muscles. He is a mime and he is incredible to watch.

Now try moving your fingers and toes in the same small way. When you set the intention to move, your muscles respond in microscopic ways. They actually get ready to move before any visible movement is made. First feel the readiness to move, and then move the particular muscle and joint you are using in very small increments in every direction it can go. I have spent more than an hour moving every joint in one hand in every possible way. It's an incredibly relaxing and centering thing to do.

Once you have learned to move in micro-movements, gradually get larger. Wriggle your toes. Shift your weight from one foot to the other. Make circles with one heel at a time. Make circles with one knee at a time. Make some pelvic circles. Tighten one buttock and then the other. Tilt your pelvis by moving your belly forward and back. Then move your ribs in a circle. Shrug your shoulders up toward your ears and let them go. Move your shoulders in circles. Move your wrists and elbows in circles. Move your neck and head in slow, gentle circles. Look down at the floor and up at the ceiling. Look behind you to the right and the left, first with your neck, then with your upper body, and then turning your whole body from your feet.

What you are doing is relearning to wriggle. When we were impatient children, our wriggling was a sign of repressing larger movements that we were not allowed to make. This time it is our *intention* to make small movements only. Intend the movements to pull your attention back from wherever in the past or future it is wandering, to your body, right now in this moment. This will remind you that you have a body at times when you previously forgot. During your normal working day, when you are caught up in your mind, it is good to check in now and then with your body.

When I was first learning the computer in order to write this book, I was very tense and stiff. It was a big change in my life to sit on a chair in one place for any length of time. I was also computer-phobic, which added to my tension. After a couple of days of aches and pains, I came back to my body and realized I needed to wriggle and stretch and let go of mental work at least every half hour. Try it. It will enhance both your productivity and aliveness. If you feel a need to have a full stretch when you become present in your body, then do so. Stretch to the ceiling and then bend down to your toes. Turn sideways from your waist and then stretch out to the side. Make big hula circles with your hips.

Try stretching while waiting in line at the grocery store. Whenever I stretch anywhere, people look at me with approval or envy. Often they will comment and sometimes they will even join in. There is something so luxurious about a full stretch. I think that is why people don't do it very often. It feels too good to do in public. If you are at a board meeting, stick with the micro-movements. No one will notice and it will relieve the tension and the tedium.

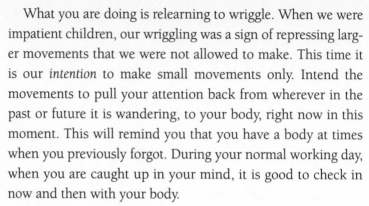

Movements … pull your attention back from wherever in the past or future it is wandering, to your body, right now in this moment.

Sitting

Sitting on chairs is cruel and unusual punishment for your body. Also, sitting for long periods in a chair is the worst thing

you can do to your back. There is more pressure on your vertebrae while sitting than while doing hard physical labor. In
native cultures, most people squat, kneel, or sit cross-legged on
the floor, and back problems are rare. Just getting up and down
from the floor keeps them healthy.

Right now, see if you can squat easily with your feet fully
on the floor. Moshe Feldenkrais used to say that this was a
sign of good muscular condition and flexibility. When I started my classes, I was surprised by how many people could not
squat and could not get up and down from a lying position
on the floor. It certainly is true about muscular strength and
flexibility that if you don't use it you lose it. We are restricting our ability to deal with crisis in our lives when our movement is limited in such a way. Ideally, we should be able to
move quickly in any direction—up, down, forward, back,
and sideways.

We learned Judo rolls in Feldenkrais training, and later, one
of the trainees fell off his bike going down a very steep hill. He
automatically rolled right over as he fell and landed on his feet
with no injuries, like an acrobat. He was sure he would have
been seriously injured without the new learning.

My mother has severe osteoporosis and has fallen occa-
sionally and hurt her back. She has fractures in every vertebra, according to the X-rays, and yet she walks normally,
takes care of herself, and has a full life. The only noticeable
difference is that she is getting shorter all the time. When her
back hurts, she moves in ways we have devised that hurt her
less. Finding a way for her to crawl back to bed would have
been funny if she hadn't been in so much pain. We tried
everything. The cycle of pain and stiffness is a very vicious
circle. If you have pain, you stiffen up; if you stiffen up, you
have more pain. The longer Mother spends sitting during the
day instead of moving about, cooking, shopping, and gardening, the stiffer she gets. The increasing amount of time
spent sitting nowadays in this culture adds enormously to the
epidemic of back problems.

Another problem caused primarily by too much sitting is the loss of bladder control I mentioned in Chapter Eight. If our chairs are usually supporting all of the organs of our lower body, the muscles of the perineum give up their work of holding them all in place. If you have a problem with bladder control when you sneeze, cough, or laugh, take heed of the warning signals.

Besides doing the exercises in Chapter Eight, the most helpful thing I have found is to get a small rebounder. They are mini trampolines, and the gentle bouncing works to strengthen all the muscles in the pelvic floor. I have one beside my desk and I love it. Jumping up and down to one or two favorite songs reawakens my body, shakes the cobwebs out of my brain, and helps all my internal organs function better. It is the best quick exercise break I know, and rebounders are very inexpensive. There should be one in every office.

When you start bouncing, you may find that you have to stop and go to the bathroom at almost every bounce at first. Start out with a very small movement of raising your heels only, so that both feet are always on the mat, and graduate up to jumping and jogging. Within a week, your muscles will have strengthened noticeably.

If you *have* to sit for long periods of time at work, remind yourself to get up and walk around and stretch every half-hour. Even as you are sitting you can get into the habit of bending and arching your spine. Fold your spine by bringing your chin toward your thighs and then look up toward the ceiling, arching your spine as much as is comfortable. Do the same bending and arching movement some more, but orient your body to the right a few times, and then to the left. Can you feel each vertebra along your spine joining in one at a time, or are you moving in three chunks? The more often you do this, the more articulated your spine will feel. Finish up with some pelvic circles while sitting in your chair.

Stretch your spine when you get up in the morning by sitting on the edge of the bed and making all of these movements.

The pelvic circles especially will free up your spine for the day ahead. If you wake up stiff, make very small and slow circles at first.

Instead of sitting on chairs and couches at home, try sitting on the floor for a week. You could also try squatting to watch television and see how long you can be comfortable in this position. I often sit on the floor because I am freer to move from there. You can roll around and bend and stretch in all kinds of ways that are impossible in a chair. You may be stiff the first day, but by the end of the week you will almost certainly feel looser and more flexible.

It would be hard to do most of our jobs while squatting, unfortunately, so the best way to sit at your desk is with both feet planted firmly on the floor. In that position, your spine can be erect with its natural curves and there are four points of support—your two feet and your two *sitz* bones. If you sit far back in your chair and lean on the backrest, you are giving up the task of supporting your body with your spine. The chair takes over the job. When you are relaxing completely, that is fine, but when you are working it is not a good idea.

When you lean on the back of your chair and extend your arms to work—writing, typing, etc.—you develop shoulder stiffness and tension. We are designed to move from the strong muscles of the pelvis and feet, and to use the articulation of all of the vertebrae. By constraining this area in the chair, we cause our neck and shoulders to do more work than they were designed to do.

There is no perfect ergonomic chair on the market that will negate the necessity to move and to wriggle. Actually, it is better to change chairs often, just as it is better for your feet to change shoes during the day. There is no one perfect position we can settle into and be safe. From the perspective of design, we were not well-designed for a sedentary lifestyle at all. We were designed to move and then to rest completely between movements.

Circular Movements

Many of the movements we learned in physical education class are very straight-line in design—jumping jacks, for example. When we use circular motions, with our spine as the axis, our movements are more natural and easier on the body. Imagine a dancer in your mind and see all the circular movements common to most dance forms. When you are moving through your daily tasks alone, pretend you are a dancer. Make your movements bigger, rounder, more graceful. Reach with your whole body from your toes instead of from your overworked shoulders. Bend all the way down, making sure not to lock the knees, whenever you need to bend.

Imagine a flow of movement instead of jerky, short, sudden moves. Put on some music and see how flowing you can be. Notice if you have a tendency to use your neck alone whenever you need to look at something to the side or behind you. Turn your whole body instead. We get so accustomed to overworking our arms, legs, and neck, and leaving our trunk rigid. Our spines are articulated like a bicycle chain; they turn, they bend, they stretch.

While you are walking around the house, think tall and light, and incorporate a few leaps and jumps and runs into your day. It is always good to have those skills available. My sister, Diane, was visiting me from England a few years ago and we were crossing a street with cars waiting when the "Don't walk" sign came on. Naturally I started to run, but when I called out to her to do the same, she walked at her normal pace. She said, "I don't run for anything" in a disapproving tone as if she were way too old for that kind of silly behavior. She was totally rigid and not yet fifty.

It was frightening to me how easily we could make a virtue out of being stiff and tight. I made up my mind right then that I would run and jump and skip and climb trees until I died. Not all the time, of course, but often enough so I wouldn't forget how. We have to be willing to be childlike on occasion to remember the pure joy of just being in our body, playing at life. We get too serious about being grownups. It's just a role we play. We don't have to lose ourselves in it. So put away all your chairs, roll around on the floor, and wriggle a lot. Your spine, neck, shoulders and, in fact, your whole body will be grateful.

Explorations for the Week

✳   Wake up your spine in the morning by stretching on the edge of your bed.

✳   Gradually incorporate more small movements into your daily life.

✳   Notice when you are caught up in a mental activity and see if you can split your awareness so that you are attuned to your body comfort while you are doing mind work. This sounds like a small thing, but actually it is huge. Be patient with yourself.

✳   Sit on the floor as much as possible.

✳   Try all the movements described in the chapter until you start to become involved in the exploration with a sense of curiosity. Then make up a million more.

✳   Wherever you are, WRIGGLE!

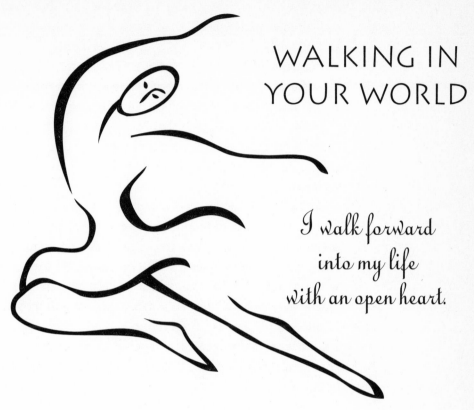

Chapter Eleven

WALKING IN YOUR WORLD

*I walk forward
into my life
with an open heart.*

To walk with freedom and grace in our world demands both muscular, mechanical skills and a psychological and spiritual connection with that world. We are the first member of the animal kingdom to choose to walk erect. By doing so we expose our soft bellies, genitals, and hearts to the rest of the world and to each other. This is a very vulnerable position. To walk forward confidently, we need to feel safe within our vulnerability.

How many people do you know who have a walk that telegraphs peace and personal power to all who see it? It's rare, isn't it? Usually it comes with the self-acceptance of maturity, if at all. That kind of confidence is also environment-specific for most of us. We will walk more freely in our own home territory than in a strange place. There is, however, a sense of safety and centeredness that we can learn to carry within us.

Einstein said that you could divide people into two groups—those for whom the world is a safe place and those for whom it is not. That personal sense of safety comes from the acknowledgment of our connections, both to the Universe and to each other. If we see most of the people in our world as well-loved sisters, brothers, and friends, we can negotiate for our needs with ease.

It is when we feel we have potential adversaries or enemies in the environment around us that we lack trust and hold our breath and tighten up. We retreat to a small safety zone in our minds somewhere and leave our bodies alone out there in the world to take care of themselves as best they can. This is when we become clumsy and uncoordinated and move like puppets. It is a very clear indication of our mental state when we move in this way. Most accidents happen when we are completely entangled in our mental processes and not in our bodies at all.

Taking all of these factors into account, walking becomes a complex topic. I will divide the movements into segments for you to notice and examine. I have included certain practical suggestions that can lead to better health and range of motion in your entire body. Underlying all of them are the psychological implications of the movements themselves, the personal history of your very particular way of walking in your world. It is impossible to separate the two. By walking differently we become different.

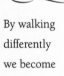

By walking differently we become different.

Moshe Feldenkrais believed that learning to move in a new, effortless way would change our lives completely. That was certainly true for me. Here is just one small example. I had a pattern of locking my knees that I was unaware of. I just knew that I couldn't learn to ice skate or ski or do anything that required balance. I felt inadequate because of that. It was a limitation in my self-image. During my Feldenkrais training,

I had a hands-on session of Functional Integration and my knees became more pliant. It was hard to explain, but they just didn't need to lock anymore. As I walked in this new way, I recaptured memories of my childhood that had been locked in my cells.

As a toddler, whenever I got to my feet my older sister would push me down. I tried to hold on to the floor by curling my toes under and locking my knees. This was the opposite of useful because locked knees make us more unstable, but what does a baby know about body mechanics? So many of our decisions to be, to move, to act in a certain way, are made before we have any logical thought processes operating. We move toward pleasure and away from pain in the natural way of kittens, and make decisions that often last a lifetime.

When I was able to let go of locking my knees in response to stress, I moved into a bigger version of who I was. I became more fully the person I was born to be. In the process of moving in a new way, you may discover for yourself where your limitations began.

Whether you remember the specific details is not important. We have all been guided into a very limited path of expression by our socialization. Most of the time we seem locked into either blind acceptance or resistance to our early role models. For all of us, there are so many paths not taken. By learning to move differently, we discover choices that we never before imagined were available to us.

Body Posture

Let's check your habitual posture or state of alignment. Stand as you would while waiting in line and notice yourself from your toes to your head, as completely as possible.

Now stand with your feet apart, the same width as your hips, so that your feet are directly underneath you. Balance evenly between them with your knees unlocked and your spine straight. Let your arms hang freely at your sides. Your head and eyes face the horizon. Breathe deeply into your belly. How do you feel? This direct, forward-facing position is very exposed, isn't it? We rarely stand like this. We normally shift our weight or do something with our arms to cover our exposed frontal surfaces.

From this balanced position, gradually round your upper back so your shoulders slump forward. Feel your knees bend a little and your neck compress and let your eyes drop to the floor ahead of you. Your arms will hang in front of your thighs. How do you feel now? Are you depressed yet? Who does this remind you of? Walk around like this and notice if your arms can swing. Do you drag your feet? Do you stare at the floor ahead?

This is the home position of someone who is saying NO to life. It is also a common position of elderly people. This is not a necessary posture of old age. We are choosing how we look at eighty by our movement patterns all our lives and by our daily reactions to life's inevitable sorrows and disappointments.

Come back to the balanced position and breathe deeply. Now put your finger on your breastbone between your breasts and push that part of you up and out. Your back will arch, your knees will start to lock, your buttocks will tighten, your chin will come forward, and your arms will hang behind your thighs. Your hands may tend to clench into fists. Your shoulder blades will come closer to your spine. How do you feel? Who does this remind you of? Stride around like this for a while. Get into it, especially if this body posture is completely foreign to you.

This is the home position of someone with an aggressive approach to life. They are using muscular armor to hide their vulnerability. Their body language says, "Don't mess with me." Underneath that they are usually saying, "I'm scared and confused so I'm trying to look tough."

Come back to your own habitual posture. Where does it fall on this huge range? What are you saying to the world? There are endless variations:

I am friendly or leave me alone.

I am better than you or pity me.

I had a client who stood before me when we met with her hands clasped in front of her, one foot leaning on the other and her head bent down a little so that she was looking up at me with her eyes. She had a neck problem that was persistent and could not be diagnosed. No wonder!

Try that position for yourself. It is the position of a child in a world of unreliable adults. After changing her way of standing, walking, and moving, she started to reclaim her power. She is more assertive now and no longer sees almost everyone in the guise of an authority figure. She was even able to be open and firm with a family member who had previously abused her. We cannot change our past, but with movement we can create choice in our present.

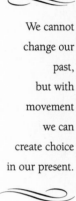

We cannot change our past, but with movement we can create choice in our present.

Feet

Now we will start back at the bottom, with our feet. Our feet are miraculous. They are designed to move. They have twenty-six bones and thirty-one joints. They are not designed for high-heeled shoes or for the flat, hard surfaces we encounter all day long. In Africa and the Ancient Americas, certain tribes could run all day on uneven terrain without shoes and without tiring. The best thing you can do for your feet is to take off your shoes as often as possible and walk barefoot on uneven surfaces. I grew up in a seaside town with a pebble beach and we locals always took malicious pleasure in watching tourists trying to walk on the pebbles. We could run on them easily, from much practice; maybe that is why my feet are so healthy today.

Many of my clients have extremely sensitive feet that act as if they have only two joints. It is hard to persuade these clients to walk barefoot, even on a soft rug; but without full utilization of all the joints of our feet, there is no way for us to move freely.

The second thing you can do to benefit your feet is to move them in every way you can think of, both on and off the ground. Turn, twist, bend, stretch, and rotate. When you are sitting reading or watching television, allow your feet to explore their possibilities. If you have ever been in a small boat, you will remember how unstable you felt at first with the movement of the water beneath your feet, and how quickly you adjusted to it. In fact, if you are in a boat for long, it is coming back on shore that feels strange.

My son, Tim, had something wrong with his feet as a child and was prescribed plastic supports for his shoes. They didn't improve anything. Then he took up surfing, which is an intricate dance between your feet and the ocean, and his feet never bothered him again.

Walk around for a while without shoes and feel how your feet contact the floor. Walk on the inside of your feet and notice what that does to your knees. Then try walking on the outside edge of your feet. Notice that even a small inward or outward slant to your feet will put your knees and hips out of alignment.

Stop walking on the floor as if it were just a dead surface and walk as if you were walking on the earth. Feel the energy of the earth rise up to support you. Make walking an interaction between you and the earth, no matter how many layers of concrete there are between you. Have you ever walked on a floating bridge? There is a dynamic interaction between your feet and the water. Imagine that the earth interacts with your feet in the same way, but more subtly.

Walking with connection to the earth gives us power. If you have been doing the Heaven and Earth breath regularly, you will have experienced that by now. If you press into the earth more with the balls of your feet so that your feet bend at each step, you will be able to walk longer with less fatigue. When I walk on the beach with a friend and we are talking, my awareness is focused on my mind and my feet get tired. When I am present in my body and pushing off of the balls of my feet at each step, I can walk for miles.

Hamstrings

Our hamstrings are the strong muscles at the back of our legs that are supposed to do most of the work of walking. By the time we are thirty, many of us have learned how to ooze along somehow without activating them. Stand with your feet hip-width apart and push into the ground with the ball of your left foot; your heel will rise slightly. Notice the motion traveling up your leg and into your behind. The harder you push, the more of your powerful walking muscles get involved. Try the right foot.

Walk around and allow these muscles—the hamstrings and the gluteal muscles of your buttocks—to spring into action at each step. Tighten them consciously at first. You may look like those men who do walking races. You will either get taller at each step or move forward faster. Practice until you can walk with or without the work of these muscles and know how different it feels. When you have to walk a long way or you are in a hurry, actively involve these muscles. Your bottom will become firmer as a side benefit from walking in this way. Your hips will also rotate more, which will be good for your lower back.

Hips

I am not including a section on knees because problems with the knees do not generally originate there, except in the case of accidental injuries. Most knee problems originate in the hips or the feet. For women of my mother's generation, hip and knee replacement surgeries are becoming commonplace, and I have been wondering whether we baby-boomers will be the same. There is a much greater awareness of the value of exercise now, but overall, our lives are more sedentary than ever. Also, many of us have all the equipment to exercise and the perfect clothes, but we still lack the will-power to work out regularly.

A huge factor in the wear on hip joints that makes a hip replacement necessary is poor body alignment. I am sorry to say that, in general, my age group seems to have even worse alignment than my mother's. The number of children with poor alignment is also increasing enormously as so many kids sit in front of televisions or Nintendos® instead of moving around playing. New plastic joints could become the norm.

The problem is that if the misalignment is not corrected, the new joints will also wear out. Some kind of re-aligning bodywork should be mandatory for women who have had replacement surgery. Physical therapy gets them walking again, but that is not enough; they have to be walking in a whole new way. For myself, I am hoping that if I move throughout my day with awareness and have good movement patterns in everything I do, I will be able to avoid deterioration in my joints.

Our hips are ball and socket joints. A lot of women move as if they don't know that. They act as if their hip joints are hinge joints like their knees. Stand up and hold onto something lightly for support and put your finger on your hip joint. It is located in the middle of the crease between your crotch and your hip-bone. Now bend your knee like a hinge and then bring your bent knee up toward your chest. That action uses your hip joint like a hinge.

Now take your knee in circles in every direction that is comfortable—side, up, down, back. You can do that only because your hip is a ball and socket joint. It's a miraculous piece of engineering and makes the wonder and beauty of dance possible.

Walk around for a while without allowing your hip joint to rotate. Your whole trunk must face forward and your hip joints will act like your knee joints. This is the walk of the wooden soldier or of a woman who has been raised to keep her bottom still as she walks. I am sure that this restriction in walking has a lot to do with the many hip problems experienced by my mother's generation. In Italy and France, women walk in a sensuous, hip-swinging way and hip replacement surgeries are uncommon.

Now walk letting your bottom move freely. In fact, exaggerate, walk like a movie star. Wiggle that behind. Notice how your hips are rotating beautifully. Notice how freely your upper body moves and your arms swing. This is a walk that involves more of you. It is more healthy in general. Tone down the wiggle until you can still feel the rotation in your hips, but it is discreet enough for your taste. Actually it is a pleasure to see people walk with their hips moving freely, and it doesn't look as provocative as it feels at first.

I have taught men this walk also and they have incorporated it into their own style without any problem. If you have ever been to Italy, you probably noticed that Italian men move their hips while walking as much as the women. Walking in this way makes us more aware of our genital area and reminds us that we are sexual beings. It is an echo of our Puritan past and patriarchal dominance that restricts this natural, healthy, enjoyable way to walk.

Your Leading Edge

The next time you are hurrying along with your mind going at a faster clip than your feet, notice what part of your body seems to be leading the rest. I used to catch myself leaning far forward like a speedskater and bustling here and there as if my mind were dragging my body along. It isn't efficient. If you are in a hurry, push off with the balls of your feet, activate your most powerful muscles, and stay in your body. You will get where you are going even sooner and more safely.

If you imagine a string tied to your belly button and someone pulling on the string as you walk, you will be leading your movement from a good place of balance. Don't stick your belly out, they aren't pulling the string that hard. Center your attention at that point as you walk and the self-confidence we were talking about at the beginning of the chapter will start to kick in. This is the point of Chi in martial arts, and it is the point around which we can rotate in any direction. It is our physical center. The powerful muscles of the pelvis and lower back are all working in harmony, leaving your upper body free to do other work.

When I see people power walking for exercise, pumping away with their arms and upper body, holding visible tension in their shoulders and neck, leaning forward and gritting their teeth, I want to beg them to stop. Let your feet, legs, and the powerful muscles in your bottom do your walking and let every muscle above them be loose and free and along for the ride. Your arms will swing freely by themselves if your hips are rotating and your lower back is moving. There is no need for tension in your shoulders or neck as you walk. A good test of a healthy walk is the ability to leap into the air freely at any time without any planning or preparation.

Explorations for the Week

* Practice walking:
  Keep your feet flexible and push off from the earth.
  Rotate those hips.
  Lead from your belly.
  Let your legs do the work.

Pretty soon you will be walking so freely that you will leap into the air and spin and turn just for the sheer joy of it. Being in a body that can move is a pleasure beyond reckoning. We lose it so gradually, if we ever had it, that we never mourn the loss. Regain that pleasure for yourself right now. You have to walk around anyway, you may as well delight in it.

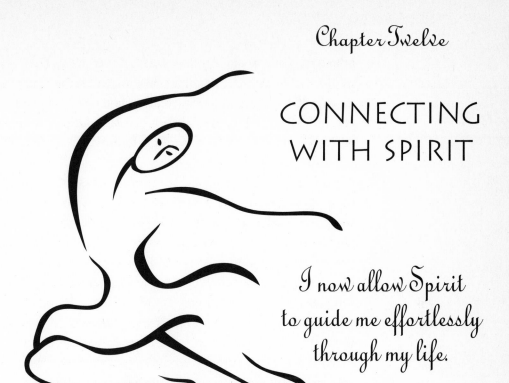

Chapter Twelve

CONNECTING WITH SPIRIT

*I now allow Spirit
to guide me effortlessly
through my life.*

I cannot imagine moving through my days without access to my Inner Wisdom, my Higher Self, and Spirit. Without them I would feel small and lost. I don't like definitions. They box things in and deny the ability to move and change; but I will try to define what these terms mean to me in *this* moment, at *this* stage of my life.

For me, Inner Wisdom refers to the small voice within that tells me when I am centered and on track in my life and when I am not. It is the little sense of discomfort I get when I am about to make a mistake. It is the desire that prods me to go somewhere or do something that turns out later to be a necessary step on my path.

My ego and personality levels want what they want, and they want it NOW. Without my Inner Wisdom to balance me, I go rushing off in pursuit of pleasure only to find that it doesn't satisfy me. My Inner Wisdom has access to information from other levels of reality. It is responsible for my flashes of insight and intuition.

My Higher Self is a personal guide. She speaks only with the voice of deep wisdom and never leads me astray. She loves me completely and unconditionally. She is the larger space within me that sees my life unfolding and knows I am on my path toward fulfilling my mission in life as best I can. She also knows that whatever emotion I feel in this particular moment will pass, and that is a truth my ego often forgets. In many religions it is said that we are all gods and goddesses. My Higher Self is the part of me that is closest to realizing that goal.

Spirit is the connection with the larger Universe of which I am a necessary and unique part. I am a drop of water and Spirit is the ocean, limitless and boundless. It is from the place of Spirit that I can heal and see other people clearly, and it is my connection with Spirit that gives me the strength to let go of something I love when I need to.

Meeting Your Higher Self

I am going to start with a visualization exercise designed to help you meet your Higher Self so that you can experience it for yourself, if you haven't already. You can either record the instructions in your own voice or have someone read them to you with feeling. Make sure you read slowly enough to complete the actions, pausing when necessary.

People have often told me that they are not good at visualization or imagining things. It turns out that they expect to get a clear image on the inside of the eyelids as if they were running a video inside their head. No one I know sees images in quite that way. Think of a purple elephant. Most people do not get a clear picture, but see it more like a dream, where trying to hold on makes it slip away. It is as if the file in our brain for purple and the file for elephant are both activated at the same time but the resulting image doesn't go through our visual apparatus.

Think of a lemon. Think of a hug. Now close your eyes and imagine a house burning down. Was it a big house? Was it a Victorian? Probably yours was not, but mine was. You are looking with your inner eyes. Change your expectations of visualization from an eyelid video to a dreamlike awareness and your contentment with the process will improve enormously.

Lie down on the floor or sit very comfortably and close your eyes. Breathe deeply into your belly and relax every part of your body, starting with your toes and working up to your forehead. Take all the time you need.

> *You are walking alone in a grassy meadow in the spring sunshine. There are flowers everywhere and the birds are singing all around. You can smell the crushed grasses and flowers as you walk and a feeling of complete peace and well-being comes over you. You feel at one with the Universe and you raise your arms to the sky and give thanks for the beauty of the day.*
>
> *You keep walking and catch sight of a beautiful building in the distance. You immediately know that it is a sacred temple and you are irresistibly drawn toward it. As you walk closer, you realize that there is a deep ravine between the meadow and the building, and you stand at the top not knowing how to cross. You look toward the left and notice some rough steps cut into a path leading down to the bottom of the ravine and you know that they were carved by women like yourself who have been here before you. You count the steps as you go down, deeper and deeper. It gets darker as you go deeper out of the sunlight, but you feel something pulling you forward, and finally you reach the bottom.*
>
> *At the bottom of the steps there is a stream and you wade across in the shallow water. When you get close to*

the other side, you see a deeper pool and a sparkle in the sunshine catches your eye. You slip out of your clothes and plunge into the warm pool. You pick up a beautiful, shining crystal from the depths and hold it to your heart.

On a rock beside the first step leading up to the temple there is a special robe waiting just for you, and you put it on and start the upward climb. Every step brings you closer to the top and you have a deep inner knowing that someone is waiting for you there who has loved you always. Finally you are at the top and you walk forward to the entrance. You stop for a moment on the threshold to center yourself, holding the crystal at your heart, and then you move into the dim room lit with shafts of sunlight from the high arched windows. The light falls softly onto an altar and you move toward it.

On the altar is a large crystal bowl full of water, and a voice within you says, "Look within to find the one you seek." You eagerly look into the water and see your own face reflected there, and for a moment you are disappointed. But as you look deeper into the eyes looking back at you from the water, you see a wisdom and an inner beauty that you didn't know you had. You gaze deeper and deeper and the image changes slowly until the face looking back at you is infinitely wise and infinitely loving, and your own voice says, "Welcome home."

The voice asks you if you have a question to ask of your Higher Self. You speak of what has been most on your mind and wait for the answer to come back to you. You treasure this wisdom from the deeper part of yourself and ask how you can meet her again when you need her. She says that she is always there for you and will come and speak with you whenever you open to her. You decide on a signal that will show you are ready to listen to your deepest wisdom.

The time has come for you to leave so, with your heart full of appreciation, you place upon the altar the crystal that you found in the pool. You move back out into the sunlight feeling new and vibrantly alive, happy as a child to have seen the one who has walked beside you for so long. You retrace your path down to the stream and change back into your own clothes. Then you cross the stream and with a light heart climb up the steps into the bird songs and flowers of the meadow. The music of nature gradually fades away and you return to the awareness of your body in the room, keeping the lightness and joy and the sense of homecoming with you as you open your eyes.

If you are in doubt at any time whether the voice inside you is the voice of your Inner Wisdom or the voice of your ego, you can signal your Higher Self in the way you chose at the temple, and she will tell you. Any small ritual will call up her presence. You could sit in the lotus position for an hour or you could jump in the air while clapping your hands. She doesn't care what you do. She is always there for you and will answer any call. I used to ignore what my Higher Self said if it didn't fit what I wanted to hear, but I have learned over time that she sees a larger picture of my beingness than I do. I trust her completely.

Direct Connection with Spirit

It is one of the major benefits of being born into a female body that women can connect directly with Spirit. It is part of our genetic heritage. There are many differences between men and women in the physiology and chemical makeup of the brain. The part of our brain that enables the right and left hemispheres to communicate is the corpus callosum. This part of the brain is forty percent larger in women than in men, and this difference enables women to balance the logical, rational mode of the left brain with the spatial, intuitive mode of the right brain.

It is one of the major benefits of being born into a female body that women can connect directly with Spirit.

In my opinion, it is because men have difficulty in connecting with Spirit directly that most religions in the world are set up and controlled by men. They have the dogma, we have direct experience. Women don't need a cathedral, a prescribed ritual, a designated intermediary, or a long list of rules. What works for each of us will be different according to our life pattern and preferences. Whatever gives you bliss in your life will bring you Home.

One quick and easy way for me to access Spirit is the Heaven and Earth breath. I do it at the beginning of meditation. I used to sit in meditation more often, but I find myself drifting away from the practice of sitting still. I would rather garden or walk or move as a spiritual practice. When I do sit, I first clearly state what I want to be and do in my life and my willingness to do the work involved; then I thank my angels and guides and allow appreciation to flood through me; and then I just sit. I watch my breath to keep my mind quiet. Sometimes I get blissed out and sometimes I get bored.

Being in nature is one of my most well-worn paths to bliss. If I am off-center or upset, I go for a walk on the beach or sit with my back against a tree. I have a deep need for that kind of contact and I get crabby without it. I have to go to the redwood forest for a few days once in a while to get back my perspective on this crazy world. I put my whole body up against the thick bark of a thousand-year-old tree and I feel in my cells how nature endures and prevails.

There are places above Big Sur where you can find the remains of old homesteads, just the foundations. Grass and brush have almost recovered their places, sneaking into all the nooks and crannies and patiently tearing down what mankind has built.

Nature makes me feel humble, and yet not insignificant, as if I am part of a huge plan and my small part is vitally needed. I feel more willing to do my part just as every tree and blade of grass does theirs. I have stood alone on the shores of oceans far from home, and I've watched the waves coming in and going

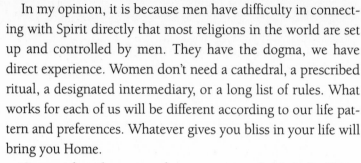

Whatever
gives you
bliss
in your life
will bring you
Home.

out, connecting me with someone I love walking on the beach back home in California.

I have always lived close to an ocean. I can get lost in the pulsation of the waves. All of nature has such ebbs and flows, the constant changing of the light and the seasons. That helps me to appreciate my own highs and lows, my fluctuating, warm and cold currents.

Art and beauty are also clear voices of the Spirit. There is special beauty in an object that is made with love. It speaks directly to your heart. Once I was in a large city in Switzerland, and I was feeling lost and scared. I was fighting with my husband and the fight felt terminal. Walking through those cold, gray streets in the middle of winter, without one leafy tree to bring me Home, I was in despair. We went into a cathedral that had some famous stained-glass windows and suddenly my breath was taken away by their beauty. I sat and let the colors rain down on me and heal my heart. It was magical. I was touched by the Divine. When I walked out of there our argument melted away under the light of pure love.

Creating anything with love is a gift to the world. We all have the power to create beauty. A wonderful meal, a poem, a drawing; we can all start somewhere. Try any art or craft that attracts you and be generous with your praise and appreciation for your efforts. Center your heart and let your Higher Self work through you. That is how I have always done my art-work. Sitting down at the potters wheel was like entering sacred space for me. My Higher Self is so infinitely creative.

I have never been able to play a musical instrument, but for many people music is a true path to Spirit. Even listening to certain music moves your energy into higher chakras. Pachelbel's *Canon* never fails to transport me to another realm. Chanting is also something that can take us very deep, and anyone can do it, although it works better in a group. Drumming is getting to be a popular way in our culture to access altered states.

And, of course, music brings us into movement, ecstatic movement. Most primitive cultures use dance or movement of some kind to bring them to an experience of the Divine. In our own country the Shakers did the same. What wonderful lives they had, such peace and simplicity and order, and then releasing into spiritual ecstasy by moving.

It is only on writing this chapter that I realize how many ways I have to make my connection with the larger Universe. When I am healing with energy I step deeply into Spirit. No matter how I feel before a session, I am also healed by the end of it. Any form of giving can have that effect for me. Giving anything from the heart can bring us Home.

A woman in my spiritual group said that certain scents connect her with Spirit. We all collected herbs and sweet-smelling flowers from the garden for someone who was going to court for a legal battle. We imbued the little bundle with our loving energy so that she could hold it in her hand and smell it and remember that she was not alone.

Ritual

Moments
of joy
and moments
of sorrow
should be
marked
amongst us ...

It is no accident that all ancient and primitive cultures, without exception, devised rituals to contact the Divine. It is a great loss to women that our rituals have been forgotten. Think how valuable it would be to have some open acknowledgment of a relationship's end. If a loved one dies, we have a right to mourn. If a lover leaves us or we leave them, we feel as much pain but we have no receptacle for our grief. We have no ashes to scatter and no body to bury. Even normal, healthy losses, like a child going off to college, are unmarked.

A ritual is the process of marking an event that is significant to us. It is a marker stone on our journey through life. Moments of joy and moments of sorrow should be marked amongst us, and the presence of Spirit could be invoked for comfort.

Think of the rituals you have in your family. Are they the same as you had as a child? Most of our rituals are around celebration times—weddings, births, holidays. Have you made up any rituals for your children on the spur of the moment? Children love rituals. They demand repetition. You just have to do something twice with a child and they say, "We *have* to do it. We *always* do that."

Nowadays we have allowed gift giving and food sharing to take over as our ritual, to say what we cannot say in words. A few years ago, I started creating rituals, making them up as I went along. We made up a ritual for the daughter of a friend on her first menstruation and a wonderful blessing circle for a new baby. For the baby we offered a gift from our hearts, a quality we wished for her to express in her life. The variety was creative and surprising.

I perform a ritual on the full moon to thank the moon that has passed and to bless the month to come. I bless the new plants I put in my garden and invoke the flower spirits to care for them. Little things, but they enrich my life. Ritual used to be a private thing for me. So many people are embarrassed by it. It feels strange and weird at first. Now it is becoming popular and I am often asked to lead a ritual or a blessing or a ceremony. It doesn't matter what you call it. You are invoking Spirit to commemorate an event in your life and Spirit is always blissfully happy to respond.

Spiritual Groups

I am in a spiritual group of women. We have been meeting for a year now and it is a great blessing in my life. We meet every other Sunday morning and we do different things each time. We have done guided visualizations, healing with energy, working with dreams, writing, rituals for various occasions, and book discussions. We can always think of something to do that makes us leave lighter and clearer than we arrived. We don't plan far ahead so that we can be free to explore the mood of the group.

We open with a deeper version of the Heaven and Earth breath and then share how our lives have been since we last met. We laugh a lot. Mostly we support each other in bringing Spirit into our daily lives. We all value the group highly. One woman started working in Colorado and she flies back every two weeks to be with us. The group is really working for us.

The power of Spirit is magnified by joining together. Try it. Begin by mentioning to women you know that you would like to start such a group. There were fifteen of us at our first meeting and some decided that it wasn't what they wanted. Now there are usually about ten and that seems like a good number. Some women had husbands they wanted included, but most of us felt we had to come together as women alone, so a different group was started for both sexes that meets at another time. Now our group is supporting me in creating a labyrinth walk in my garden as a sacred place for ritual and inner healing.

It turns out that writing this book has become a deep, spiritual experience for me. The first draft was me. All the ideas and suggestions were there, but the flow of Spirit was lacking. It was written by my mind. I made a ritual ceremony, set the intention to help women, called in a blessing, and gave the book up to Spirit. It is amazing how it progressed after that.

It certainly is true that it is by teaching that you learn. For years, when women asked me why I wasn't teaching, I would say I wasn't ready yet. That's so left-brained. We are all teachers for each other and, with the guidance of Spirit, we can spread compassion, love, and laughter in our lives.

The power
of Spirit
is magnified
by joining
together.

Explorations for the Week

✳ Remember some family rituals from your childhood and how you felt about them.

✳ Remember a time in your childhood when you felt connected to Spirit.

✳ Remember a loss you suffered that was never acknowledged, and create a ritual to honor that loss. You can use incense, candles, flowers, water, fire. You can have a burial in the earth of your hopes and dreams. You could draw or write something and burn it. Let the part of you that knows how to do it take over.

✳ Be in nature and connect with Spirit.

✳ Connect with someone you love from the level of Spirit and see them absolutely clearly.

✳ Get in touch with the way you contact Spirit the best, your own special way. Clarify it to yourself and ritualize it so that it will be available to you even when you are in distress.

Resource List

Rodegast, Pat. *Emmanuel's Book*. New York: Bantam Books, 1987.

Douglas-Klotz, Neil. *Prayers of the Cosmos*. San Francisco: HarperCollins Publishers, 1990.

Karpinsky, Gloria D. *Where Two Worlds Touch*. New York: Ballantine Books, 1990.

Anderson, Joan Wester. *Where Miracles Happen*. Brett Books, Inc.

Mascetti, Manuela Dunn. *The Song of Eve*. New York: Fireside/ Simon & Schuster, 1990.

CONGRATULATIONS

You have finished the book. If you were doing a read-through, then it's time to start again and really do the work. If you've done the work, you have already come home to your body. Enjoy your new life. My blessing for you is to wish you joy, love, peace, comfort in your body, mind, and Spirit, and a deep connection with your Inner Wisdom and Higher Self.

INDEX

Stay in Touch. . .

Llewellyn publishes hundreds of books on your favorite subjects.

On the following pages you will find listed some books now available on related subjects. Your local bookstore stocks most of these and will stock new Llewellyn titles as they become available. We urge your patronage.

Order by Phone

Call toll-free within the U.S. and Canada, 1–800–THE MOON.
In Minnesota call **(612) 291–1970.**
We accept Visa, MasterCard, and American Express.

Order by Mail

Send the full price of your order (MN residents add 7% sales tax) in U.S. funds to:

> **Llewellyn Worldwide**
> **P.O. Box 64383, Dept. K290–9**
> **St. Paul, MN 55164–0383, U.S.A.**

Postage and Handling

- $4.00 for orders $15.00 and under
- $5.00 for orders over $15.00
- No charge for orders over $100.00

We ship UPS in the continental United States. We cannot ship to P.O. boxes. Orders shipped to Alaska, Hawaii, Canada, Mexico, and Puerto Rico will be sent first-class mail.

International orders: Airmail—add freight equal to price of each book to the total price of order, plus $5.00 for each non-book item (audio-tapes, etc.). Surface mail—Add $1.00 per item.

Allow 4–6 weeks delivery on all orders. Postage and handling rates subject to change.

Group Discounts

We offer a 20% quantity discount to group leaders or agents. You must order a minimum of 5 copies of the same book to get our special quantity price.

Free Catalog

Get a free copy of our color catalog, *New Worlds of Mind and Spirit*. Subscribe for just $10.00 in the United States and Canada ($20.00 overseas, first-class mail). Many bookstores carry *New Worlds*—ask for it!

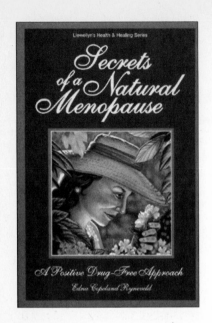

SECRETS OF A NATURAL MENOPAUSE
A Positive, Drug-Free Approach

Edna Copeland Ryneveld

Negotiate your menopause without losing your health, your sanity, or your integrity! *Secrets of a Natural Menopause* provides you with simple, natural treatments—using herbs, vitamins and minerals, foods, homeopathy, yoga, and meditation—that are safer (and cheaper) than estrogen replacement therapy.

Simply turn to the chapter describing the treatment you're interested in and look up any symptom from arthritis, depression, and hair loss to osteoporosis and varicose veins—you'll find time-honored as well as modern methods of preventing or alleviating menopausal symptoms that work, all described in plain, friendly language you won't need a medical dictionary to understand.

For years, allopathic medicine has treated menopause as a disease brought on by a deficiency of hormones instead of a perfectly natural transition. *Secrets of a Natural Menopause* will help you discover what's best for your body and empower you to take control of your own health and well-being.

1-56718-596-7, 6 x 9, 224 pp., illus., softcover $12.95

To Order by Phone: 1–800–THE MOON
Prices subject to change without notice

CREATE YOUR OWN JOY
A Guide for Transforming Your Life

Elizabeth Jean Rogers

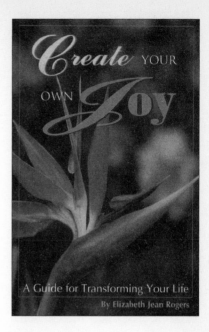

Uncover the wisdom, energy, and love of your higher self and discover the peace and joy for which you yearn! This highly structured journal-workbook is designed to guide you through the process of understanding how you create your own joy by how you choose to respond to people and situations in your life.

Each chapter offers guided meditations on overcoming blocks—such as guilt, grief, fear, and destructive behavior—that keep happiness from you; thoughtful questions to help you focus your feelings; concrete suggestions for action; and affirmations to help you define and fulfill your deepest desires and true needs. As you record your responses to the author's questions, you will transform this book into a personal expression of your own experience.

Life is too short to waste your energy on negative thoughts and emotions—use the uncomplicated, dynamic ideas in this book to get a fresh outlook on current challenges in your life, and open the door to your joyful higher self.

1-56718-354-9, 6 x 9, 240 pp., illus., softcover $10.00

To Order by Phone: 1–800–THE MOON
Prices subject to change without notice

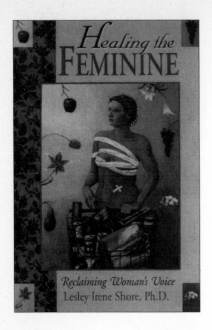

HEALING THE FEMININE
Reclaiming Woman's Voice

Lesley Irene Shore, Ph.D.

Most self-help books for women inadvertently add to women's difficulties by offering ways to battle symptoms of distress without examining the underlying causes. One of the first of its kind, *Healing the Feminine* chronicles the struggles and triumphs of a psychologist and her clients on their personal journeys to self-discovery and wholeness.

Tracing much of women's distress to society's devaluation of the feminine, Dr. Shore illustrates the need for both men and women to reclaim their hidden but vital feminine aspects. Reconnecting with the feminine entails affirming the female experience, the female body, and the female way of being. Through a variety of methods that include breathing exercises, mental imagery, and living in tune with nature, we can learn to hear our hidden "Woman's Voice" and begin the journey to wholeness and peace.

1-56718-667-X, 5¼ x 8, 208 pp., softcover   **$12.00**

To Order by Phone: 1–800–THE MOON
Prices subject to change without notice

SENSUOUS LIVING
Expand Your Sensory Awareness

Nancy Conger

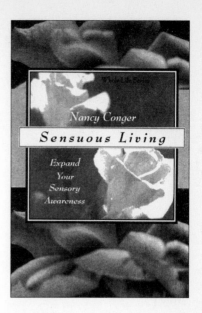

Take a wonderful journey into the most intense source of delight and pleasure humans can experience: the senses! Enjoying your sense of sight, sound, smell, taste, and touch is your birthright. Learn to treasure it with this guide to sensuous living.

Most of us revel in our senses unabashedly as children, but societal norms gradually train us to be too busy or disconnected from ourselves to savor them fully. By intentionally practicing sensuous ways of living, you can regain the art of finding beauty and holiness in simple things. This book provides activities to help you engage fully in life through your senses. Relish the touch of sun-dried sheets on your skin. Tantalize your palate with unusual foods and taste your favorites with a new awareness. Attune to tiny auditory pleasures that surround you, from the click of computer keys to raindrops hitting a window. Appreciate light, shadow, and color with an artist's eye.

Revel in the sensory symphony that surrounds you and live more fully. Practice the fun techniques in this book and heighten every moment of your life more—you're entitled!

1-56718-160-0, 6x9, 224 pp., illus., softcover $12.95

To Order by Phone: 1–800–THE MOON
Prices subject to change without notice

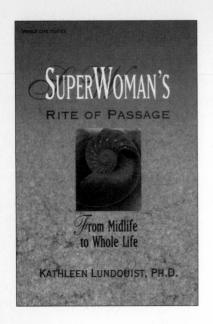

SUPERWOMAN'S RITE OF PASSAGE
From Midlife to Whole Life

Kathleen F. Lundquist, Ph.D.

Midlife transition is uniquely challenging to the "Superwoman" because her success has come too often at the expense of her feminine psyche. For women who have nurtured the more masculine aspects of their psyches for academic achievement, career recognition, and financial independence, life after forty can look grim. *Superwoman's Rite of Passage* is a workbook for high-achieving women who are entering midlife and want to emerge from this transition whole and renewed.

Superwoman's Rite of Passage transforms the challenge of midlife into an enriching personal adventure. Guide yourself through the five stages of a process called "Re-Membering," from which you birth your "Authentic Adultwoman." This process is enhanced by reflective exercises and rituals calling upon nature guides and archetypal goddesses who reaffirm the truth that "You are not alone," "Support is all around you" and "You are not going crazy." *Superwoman's Rite of Passage* is a blueprint for women searching for a sense of wholeness that's been squelched by patriarchal conditioning. Reconnect with your feminine psyche and achieve wholeness.

1-56718-447-2, 6 x 9, 240 pp., softcover $14.95

To Order by Phone: 1–800–THE MOON
Prices subject to change without notice

THE WOMEN'S BOOK OF HEALING

Diane Stein

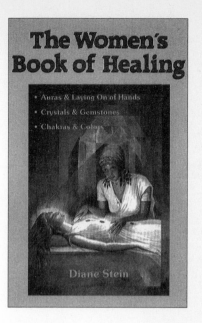

At the front of the women's spirituality movement with her previous books, Diane Stein now
helps women (and men) reclaim their natural
right to be healers. Included are exercises that
can help YOU to become a healer! Learn about
the uses of color, vibration, crystals, and gems
for healing. Learn about the auric energy field
and the Chakras.

The book teaches alternative healing theory and techniques
and combines them with crystal and gemstone healing, laying
on of stones, psychic healing, laying on of hands, chakra work
and aura work, and color therapy. It teaches beginning theory
in the aura, chakras, colors, creative visualization, meditation,
health theory, and ethics with some quantum theory. Forty-six
gemstones plus clear quartz crystals are discussed in detail,
arranged by chakras and colors.

The Women's Book of Healing is a book designed to teach basic
healing (Part I) and healing with crystals and gemstones (Part
II). Part I discusses the aura and four bodies; the chakras; basic
healing skills of creative visualization, meditation and color
work; psychic healing; and laying on of hands. Part II begins
with a chapter on clear quartz crystal, then enters gemstone
work with introductory gemstone material. The remainder of
the book discusses, in chakra-by-chakra format, specific gemstones for healing work, their properties and uses.

0-87542-759-6, 6 x 9, 352 pp., illus., softcover   **$14.95**

To Order by Phone: 1–800–THE MOON
Prices subject to change without notice

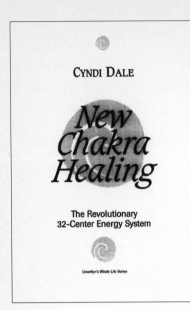

CYNDI DALE

New Chakra Healing

The Revolutionary
32-Center Energy System

Llewellyn's Whole Life Series

NEW CHAKRA HEALING
The Revolutionary 32-Center Energy System

Cyndi Dale

Break through the barriers that keep you from your true purpose with *New Chakra Healing*. This manual presents never-before-published information that makes a quantum leap in the current knowledge of the human energy centers, fields, and principles that govern the connection between the physical and spiritual realms.

By working with your full energy body, you can heal all resistance to living a successful life. The traditional seven-chakra system was just the beginning of our understanding of the holistic human. Now Cyndi Dale's research uncovers a total of 32 energy centers: 12 physically oriented chakras, and 20 energy points that exist in the spiritual plane. She also discusses auras, rays, kundalini, mana energy, karma, dharma, and cords (energetic connections between people that serve as relationship contracts). In addition, she extends chakra work to include the back of the body as well as the front, with detailed explanations on how these energy systems tie into the spine. Each chapter takes the reader on a journey through the various systems, incorporating personal experiences, practical exercises and guided meditation.

1-56718-200-3, 7 x 10, 288 pp., illus., softcover $17.95

To Order by Phone: 1–800–THE MOON
Prices subject to change without notice